Breast Cancer
Clear & Simple

All Your Questions Answered

Breast Cancer
Clear & Simple

All Your Questions Answered

Second Edition

From the Experts at the American Cancer Society

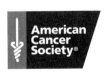

Published by the American Cancer Society
250 Williams Street NW
Atlanta, GA 30303-1002
Copyright ©2016 American Cancer Society

Printed in the United States of America
Cover design by Rikki Campbell Ogden/pixiedesign llc
Plain language review by Regan Minners, Walnutbrain Consulting
Illustrations by Samuel K. Collins, CMI, FAMI, and Amy P. Collins, FAMI

5 4 3 2   16 17 18 19 20

Library of Congress Cataloging-in-Publication Data
Names: American Cancer Society.
Title: Breast cancer clear & simple : all your questions answered / from the
    experts at the American Cancer Society.
Other titles: Breast cancer clear and simple
Description: Second edition. | Atlanta, GA : American Cancer Society,
    [2016] | Series: Clear & simple
Identifiers: LCCN 2015037215| ISBN 9781604432367 (paperback) |
    ISBN 1604432365 (paperback)
Subjects: LCSH: Breast--Cancer--Popular works. | BISAC: HEALTH &
    FITNESS / Diseases / Cancer. | HEALTH & FITNESS / Women's
    Health. | MEDICAL / Preventive Medicine.
Classification: LCC RC280.B8 B673 2016 | DDC 616.99/449--dc23 LC
    record available at http://lccn.loc.gov/2015037215

For more information about breast cancer, contact your American Cancer Society at **800-227-2345** or **cancer.org**.

Quantity discounts on bulk purchases of this book are available. Book excerpts can also be created to fit specific needs. For information, please send an e-mail to **trade.sales@cancer.org**.

For general inquiries about American Cancer Society books, send an e-mail to **acsbooks@cancer.org**.

American Cancer Society

Book Publishing

Senior Director, Journals and Book Publishing: **Esmeralda Galán Buchanan**

Managing Editor: **Rebecca Teaff, MA**

Senior Editor: **Jill Russell**

Book Publishing Manager: **Vanika Jordan, MSPub**

Editorial Assistant: **Amy Rovere**

Cancer Control Programs and Services

Senior Vice President: **Chuck Westbrook**

Managing Director, Content: **Eleni Berger**

Director, Cancer Information: **Louise Chang, MD**

Medical Editor: **Rick Alteri, MD**

Illustrations

The medical illustrations for this book were created by Samuel K. Collins, CMI, FAMI, and Amy P. Collins, FAMI, and first appeared in *Breast Cancer Journey, Third Edition*, ©American Cancer Society 2013.

List of Illustrations

Acknowledgments

Reviewers

The publisher gratefully acknowledges the following individuals who reviewed the original manuscript for *Breast Cancer Clear & Simple* and provided helpful recommendations for this second edition.

American Cancer Society

Managing Director, Mission Program Management: **Marcia Watts, MBA**

Director, Mission Delivery, Midwest Division: **Jennifer Wentzel**

Specialist, Mission Delivery, Midwest Division: **Amy Peters, MD**

American Cancer Society/Reach To Recovery® Volunteers

Sandy Ends

Cathy Hirsch, JD

Anne Abate, PhD

Contributors to the First Edition

We also wish to thank these contributors to the first edition:

Writer: **Amy Brittain**

Plain Language Writer and Editor: **Wendy Mettger, MA**

Medical Reviewer: **Terri Ades, DNP, FNP-BC, AOCN**

A Note to the Reader

Reading this book is not the same as getting medical advice from a doctor. This book may not include all possible choices, treatments, medicines, safety measures, side effects, or results associated with breast cancer. For any choices that affect your health, talk with a medical doctor who knows your health history.

This book is addressed to women with breast cancer. Breast cancer can also occur in men, but the disease is 100 times more common in women. To learn more about breast cancer in men, visit our website at **cancer.org**, or call your American Cancer Society at **800-227-2345**.

Breast Cancer Journey, Third Edition, also published by the American Cancer Society, was a major resource for this book. Specific details for information derived from *Breast Cancer Journey* are provided in references throughout the text.

Contents

Treating Your Breast Cancer

Recovering from Treatment

More Information

Introduction

About this book

It's important to know what to expect during your breast cancer treatment and recovery. We've written this book to help you—

- understand breast cancer;
- learn how it may affect you;
- learn about your treatment choices;
- face problems with money, work, or your home life;
- recover from breast cancer; and
- get your life back.

This book has answers to many common questions about breast cancer. We also suggest some questions you may ask your doctor about breast cancer and your personal treatment plan. We encourage you to discuss your treatment choices with your doctor.

How to use this book

This book is divided into two sections.

The first section takes you step-by-step through—

- **finding out** you have breast cancer—the diagnosis;
- **treating** your breast cancer; and
- **recovering** from treatment.

The second section, "More Information," gives you details about breast cancer risk and staging.

There is a lot of information in this book. Read only what you want to read right now. Use the "Contents" section at the front of the book to help you quickly find what interests you. The resource guide on pages 175–183 tells you about services for cancer patients and their families. These resources help patients and their loved ones understand cancer, manage treatment, and find all types of support for dealing with cancer. A glossary of medical terms is on pages 184–190.

Finding Out You Have Breast Cancer

What now?

You may be in shock. You may feel angry, worried, overwhelmed, hopeless, or scared. In fact, you may not know what to do. That's okay. It's normal to be upset and confused. No one wants to hear that she has breast cancer.

Don't rush.

You may feel like your cancer must be treated right now, even if you aren't sure how. But it is important to learn as much as you can about your breast cancer before making decisions about treatment. Take a few days or weeks to talk with your doctor about your options. That way, you can be sure you're making the best choices for you and your health.

What will happen to me?

Will I be okay?

Each person's cancer is different.

Most women with breast cancer are treated and recover. In fact, more than 3.5 million women in the United States have had breast cancer and are alive today.[1]

You may already know family members and friends who have had breast cancer, were treated, and went on with their lives. These examples are proof that for most women, there is life after breast cancer.

Experts are working all the time on better ways to find and treat breast cancer.

Will I lose my breast?

Most women do not lose a breast.

Doctors can often remove the cancer without removing the whole breast. They take out the cancerous lump and some of the breast tissue around the cancer. This is called lumpectomy, or breast-conserving surgery.

What if I need to have my breast removed?

Some women do need to have their whole breast removed to get all the cancer.

Removing one breast is called a mastectomy. Removing both breasts is called a double mastectomy.

It is very upsetting to lose one or both of your breasts. You will need information and support to help you cope with your loss.

Read more about lumpectomy and mastectomy on pages 40–54.

Will I be in pain?

Having cancer does not mean you have to be in pain.

If you have pain from cancer or cancer treatment, there are many ways you can feel better. You don't have to suffer through any pain you feel. Medicines and some ways of relaxing can help. Here are some suggestions:

- **Remember that controlling your cancer pain is part of your cancer treatment.**

- **Talk with your doctors about any pain you feel.** The more doctors know about your pain, the better job they can do to relieve it. Don't be afraid to talk about your pain.

- **Ask for help to treat your pain.** Getting relief from your pain can help you deal with your cancer. Being free of pain will help you stay strong so you can get through your cancer treatment.

- **Don't feel you have to choose between getting treated for cancer and getting treated for pain.** Doctors can help you with your pain while treating your cancer.

My friend had breast cancer. Will my experience be the same as hers?

Each woman with breast cancer is different.

What happens to one woman with breast cancer won't happen to all women with breast cancer. Here are a few reasons why:

- **Breast cancer affects people in different ways.** Not everyone with one type of cancer has the same experience.
- **There are different kinds of breast cancer.** They affect the body in different ways.

Doctors don't treat every breast cancer the same way. They think about your breast cancer and your health. Then they make a treatment plan for your cancer.

My loved one had another kind of cancer. Should I expect my experience to be the same as hers?

Not all cancers are the same.

You've probably known someone who has had cancer. Just because something happened to that person does not mean it will happen to you. There are several reasons for this:

- Some types of cancer can be treated more easily than other types.
- Some types of cancer and cancer treatments make people sicker than others.
- Some cancers are found when they are small and easier to treat. Others are found later, after they have been growing for a while, and are harder to treat.
- People often have other illnesses that affect how they respond to the cancer treatment.

What Is Breast Cancer?

Breast cancer is a complex disease. There are different types of breast cancer. Each type is different and needs specific treatments.

This drawing of normal breast tissue shows the 3 main components of the female breast: (1) lobules, the glands that produce milk; (2) ducts, the passages that carry the milk from the lobules to the nipple; and (3) stroma, the fatty and connective tissues surrounding the ducts and lobules.

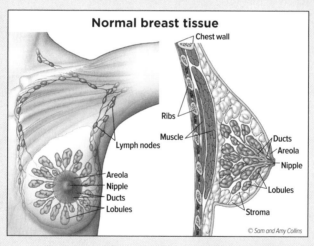

Normal breast tissue

Chest wall

Ribs

Muscle

Lymph nodes

Areola
Nipple
Ducts
Lobules

Ducts
Areola
Nipple
Lobules
Stroma

© Sam and Amy Collins

Most types of breast cancer begin in the cells that line the ducts. This is called ductal cancer. Some types begin in the cells that line the lobules. This is called lobular cancer. Only a small number of breast cancers start in the cells of the stroma of the breast.

How cancer starts

All living things, from plants to people, are made up of tiny cells. The healthy cells in your body grow, form new cells, and die when they're supposed to.

But cancer cells are not normal and don't follow the patterns they should. They don't die like other cells. They keep growing and making new cells. In the most common types of breast cancer, these cells grow out of control and form a lump called a tumor. If the cancer is around long enough, it can spread to other parts of the body.

More facts about breast cancer

- When doctors find breast cancer before it grows into a large tumor or spreads, they can treat it more easily.

- There are different types of breast cancer, and not every breast cancer grows the same way. So doctors don't treat every breast cancer the same way.

- Breast cancer happens mostly in women, but men can get breast cancer, too.

For information about different types of breast cancer, call the American Cancer Society at **800-227-2345**, or go to **cancer.org**.

Why me?

Is it my fault I have breast cancer?

No. It's not your fault.[2]

Many women want to know why they got breast cancer. Some women think they did something to cause their cancer. They may think they got breast cancer as a punishment for something they did or didn't do. Or they may think if they had done something differently, they wouldn't have gotten breast cancer. These reactions to a diagnosis are understandable, but don't blame yourself. You did not cause your breast cancer.

We don't know what makes most breast cancers start to grow. We do know that some things in a woman's life affect her chances of getting breast cancer. This is called her breast cancer risk. But even when certain factors are thought to raise a woman's chance of getting breast cancer, there's no way to know if they actually contribute to her getting it.

For more information about breast cancer risk, see pages 155–160.

If I don't feel sick, do I really have cancer?

Cancer doesn't always make you feel sick.

Some women say they can't believe they have cancer because they feel fine. It can be hard to accept that you have breast cancer when you don't feel sick. Other women may not feel quite right for a while before doctors find their breast cancer.

Cancer can grow silently for a long time before it causes problems or pain. That's why getting checked regularly for cancer is so important. The earlier cancer is found and treated, the better your chances for a long life after treatment.

How serious is my cancer?

How do the doctors know how serious my cancer is?

They first study a sample of your breast tissue.

Doctors study the breast tissue sample that was taken out during the biopsy and write a pathology report. It explains the type of breast cancer you have. It also says whether your tumor is likely to grow quickly or slowly.

Doctors use the report as a guide to help them plan how to treat your cancer. If you have surgery, the pathology report from surgery will be more detailed than the initial report.

What does "cancer grade" mean?

"Cancer grade" refers to how likely it is that your cancer will grow and spread quickly.

When doctors talk about "cancer grade," it is one way of talking about how serious your cancer is.

To decide the grade of your cancer, doctors look at your cancer cells under a microscope. They give your cancer a grade from 1 to 3. Cancer grades are described as follows:

- **grade 1,** or low grade;
- **grade 2,** or intermediate grade; and
- **grade 3,** or high grade.

A doctor will assign a grade to the cancer based on how closely the biopsy sample resembles normal breast tissue. Under a microscope, grade 1 cancer cells will look the most like healthy, normal cells. They are less likely to grow and spread quickly. Cancer cells that are grade 3 will look the most different from normal cells. They are more serious and could grow more quickly.

What does "cancer stage" mean?

"Cancer stage" tells you how much cancer there is and if the cancer has spread.

The cancer stage helps your doctor determine your treatment options and figure out what is likely to happen with your cancer.

To decide the stage of your cancer, your doctor will use the results of the physical exam and biopsy, along with results from surgery, if applicable. Other tests that might be used include a chest x-ray, mammograms of both breasts, bone scans, computed tomography (CT) scans, magnetic resonance imaging (MRI) scans, and positron emission tomography (PET) scans. (Most women won't need all of these tests.)

In cancer staging, a system of letters and numbers is used to describe the following:

- the size of your breast tumor;
- whether your cancer has grown into nearby structures (like the skin);
- whether your cancer has reached nearby lymph nodes; and
- whether your cancer has spread to other parts of your body.

See pages 161–164 for more information about cancer staging.

The doctor says my breast cancer has spread. What does that mean?

It's possible for cancer to spread to another part of the body.

Sometimes cancer cells break away from a tumor and spread to other parts of the body through the bloodstream or lymph vessels. The cancer cells can settle in other places in the body and form new tumors. When cancer cells spread to another place in the body, it is called metastasis.

Even when cancer has spread to a new place in the body, the cancer is still named after the part of the body where it started. If breast cancer spreads to the lungs, for example, it is still called breast cancer. Breast cancer is most likely to spread to the bones. Other common sites are the liver, lungs, and brain. Breast cancer can also spread to other parts of the body.[3]

Do my doctors know how well I will respond to treatment?

Your doctors can predict how likely you are to respond to treatment, but no one can be sure.

Your doctors study what has happened to other women who had breast cancer with the same stage and grade as yours, and they consider the hormone receptor and HER2 status of your breast cancer. They look at how well treatment worked for those women to better predict how well you might do with treatment.

Testing for hormone receptors in the breast tissue is an important part of evaluating breast cancer status. At the time of biopsy or surgery, the breast cancer cells are tested to see if estrogen or progesterone receptors are present. Breast cancer cells that have one or both of these receptors are considered hormone-receptor positive. About 2 of 3 breast cancers are hormone-receptor positive. These cancers tend to grow more slowly and are much more likely to respond to hormone therapy than cancers that lack these receptors.

Invasive breast cancers, or those that have spread beyond the top layer of cells in the milk ducts or lobules, should also be tested for HER2, a growth-promoting protein. Tumors containing high levels of HER2 are referred to as HER2-positive tumors. About 1 in 5 breast cancers has too much of this protein. These cancers tend to grow and spread more quickly than others. However, these cancers are also more likely to respond to drugs that target the HER2 protein.

What is meant by the word "prognosis"?

This term means what will probably happen with your cancer.

Prognosis is your outlook after your diagnosis. This includes the time during cancer treatment and afterwards. It relates to your chances of recovering from cancer and having a recurrence.

But you are not a number on a chart. You are a person. Your body will react to cancer and treatment in its own way. Just because something happened to other women with breast cancer like yours does not mean it will happen to you. And cancer treatment is getting better all the time, so numbers and charts don't always reflect the many resources that are helping women right now.

Why doesn't the doctor use the word "cure"?

Even after treatment, it's hard to know if every cancer cell is gone forever.

Most doctors use the word "remission" instead of "cure." If they say "Your cancer is in remission," this means that tests done after your treatment don't show any cancer. This is a wonderful moment for many women!

A few cancer cells might still be hidden somewhere in the body, though, and start growing later. That's why doctors don't like to use the word "cure." They can't guarantee that the cancer is completely gone, even if it's very likely that it is.

Many women recover completely from breast cancer and have no sign of any cancer in their bodies. Other women who still have evidence of cancer are able to keep it under control and live long lives.

Do I need a second opinion?

Consider getting a second opinion. It can be important to know what another doctor says about your breast cancer.[4]

You may want to get a second opinion about your diagnosis. That is, you may want to talk with other doctors about your diagnosis and the treatment plan your first doctor suggested. This way, you can feel more confident that the first doctor had the best plan, and it will help ensure that you understand all of your treatment options.

Your insurance provider might pay for a second opinion if you request it. Some insurance plans might even require that you get one. Talk with someone from your insurance company to find out what costs will be covered before you go to another doctor.

After talking with different doctors, think about what you have learned. Talk it over with friends and family members. Then choose the best treatment plan for you. Once you make that decision, it's time to start your breast cancer treatment.

Won't the first doctor be mad if I want to talk to someone else?

Most doctors will understand why you want a second opinion.

Women with breast cancer frequently seek a second opinion on their diagnosis and treatment. Wanting a second opinion doesn't mean you believe that the first doctor gave you poor treatment or advice, or that you don't trust the doctor. It means you want to explore all your options and make certain you have the right treatment plan. And getting another opinion may be required by your insurance company.

Many doctors will encourage you to talk with another doctor about your biopsy, your cancer diagnosis, and what is likely to happen. They know that your health and life are at stake. If your doctor gets mad or refuses to suggest another doctor, then you need to think about whether he or she is the right doctor for you.

? Questions

to ask the doctor who told you
about your cancer

1. What is my breast cancer grade?

2. What could this cancer grade mean for my health and my life?

3. What is the stage of my breast cancer?

4. How does my cancer stage affect which cancer treatments I should have?

5. How does my cancer stage affect my prognosis?

6. Was my breast cancer found to be hormone-receptor positive? If so, how will this impact my treatment?

7. Was my breast cancer found to be HER2 positive? If so, how will this affect my treatment?

8. Could you explain the different parts of my pathology report to me?

9. I'd like a second opinion. How do I get one?

10. Can you recommend a doctor to give me a second opinion?

11. How do I get my biopsy samples to that doctor?

12. What other tests do you think I will need?

Treating Your Breast Cancer

Who will help with my cancer treatment?

Can I choose my doctor?

You will likely be able to choose who will be in charge of your cancer treatment, although your choices might be limited based on your insurance coverage.

Talk with your primary care doctor about finding an oncologist. An oncologist is a doctor who specializes in treating people with cancer. You will want to find an oncologist who has treated a lot of women with breast cancer.

Most hospitals have several doctors who treat breast cancer. They may be experts in cancer, surgery, or radiation treatment. Your oncologist will likely oversee all your treatment.

You may have to pay more if you choose a doctor who is outside your insurance provider's network. Ask your insurance provider so you will know what will be covered.

What should I think about when choosing a doctor?

Think about what you want most from a doctor.

You will be with your oncologist for quite some time. He or she will work with you to create a treatment plan. And you will continue to see your oncologist for regular checkups for years after treatment ends. It is really important to find an oncologist you trust.

Here are some questions that may help you choose your oncologist:

- Does the doctor treat you with respect?
- Does the doctor explain things in a way you can understand?
- Does the doctor listen to your concerns and questions?
- Do you and the doctor share a common approach to your health and breast cancer treatment?
- Will you be able to reach the doctor when you have questions or need information?
- Has the doctor treated a lot of women with breast cancer like yours?

Your decision about which doctor to see may be closely tied to the hospital where he or she works.

Where will I go for treatment?

It's most likely that you will go to the hospital or outpatient clinic where your oncologist works.

Most doctors only work at certain hospitals. Find out whether the hospital where your doctor works is known for excellence in cancer care.

You can ask your oncologist and primary care doctor specific questions about treatment centers. They will help you feel comfortable about the hospital or center where you will receive care.

Who else will care for me?

There will be many people caring for you during your cancer treatment.[5]

One person on your medical team will take the lead in coordinating your care. You may be able to decide whom this person will be. Your strongest ally could be your primary care doctor, who has probably known you longer and better than the other caregivers. The medical team lead could also be your oncologist or surgeon. It should be made clear to all other team members who is in charge of your case; that person will inform the others of your progress. You will see doctors, nurses, and other medical staff trained to help women with breast cancer.

The chart on the next page shows the people who may be part of your care team. See pages 165–170 for descriptions of these team members.

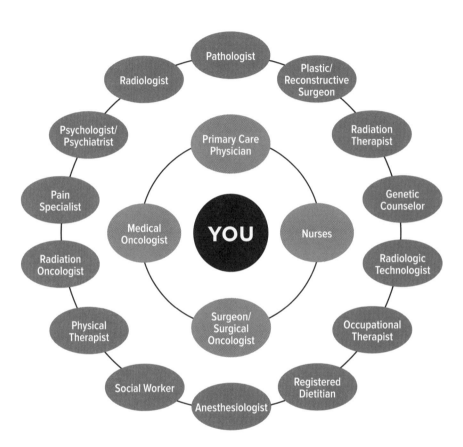

? Questions

to ask a doctor who may treat you

1. What is the exact type of breast cancer I have? How common is it?

2. Have you treated this type of breast cancer before? If so, how many patients have you treated?

3. When is your office open?

4. Who would take care of me if you were on vacation or if I needed help when the office was closed?

5. Can I bring someone to appointments with me to take notes?

6. What treatment(s) do you recommend for my breast cancer, and why?

7. At which hospital would I be treated?

8. Does this hospital treat a lot of women with breast cancer?

9. Does the hospital have the latest technology for treating breast cancer?

10. Are you willing to talk with my family members about their concerns?

11. Do you have information about breast cancer that I can take with me?

12. Where can I find more information about breast cancer?

How to Talk with Your Doctor

It's not always easy to talk with your doctor. You may feel worried, think your questions are silly, or just feel too tired to talk. Also, your doctor may be in a rush. You may get the feeling that he or she is too busy to take the time to answer your questions. All these issues can make it hard to talk with your doctor.

Here are some tips to help you feel more comfortable talking with your doctor and asking questions:

- Tell the doctor right away that you have questions.
- Have your list of questions ready.
- Understand that there are no "stupid" or "silly" questions.
- Take notes of what your doctor says.
- Have someone come with you to help ask questions and take notes.

Why ask questions?

Questions are important for these reasons:

- You need to understand what is going on.
- You should know why the doctor thinks you should have a certain test or treatment.

- You want to make sure you agree with your doctor's suggestions.

Asking questions doesn't make you a bad patient. It's your doctor's job to tell you about your cancer and what you need to do to get better.

Make sure you understand

The words that doctors and nurses use to talk about cancer can be hard to understand. They may use terms you have never heard before. If you have trouble understanding them, these tips may help:

- Ask them to explain the word.
- Ask them to draw a picture to explain the word or concept.
- Ask them to give you an example from everyday life to help explain the word.

Work as a team

The more you can talk with your doctor and get answers to your questions, the better you can work together during your breast cancer treatment. A teamwork approach will help you get good care.

What's the best way to treat my breast cancer?

What kind of treatment will I get?

There are many ways to treat breast cancer.

Your doctor will suggest a special treatment plan for you. Your plan may include one or more of the following treatments:

- Surgery
- Radiation therapy
- Chemotherapy
- Hormone therapy
- Targeted therapy
- Bone-directed therapy

How do I know whether my doctors are suggesting the best treatment?

Talk with your oncologist about what treatments have worked best for your type of breast cancer.

Ask why your doctor is suggesting certain kinds of treatment. Are these treatments the most effective for your type of breast cancer? Ask for more information about the treatment your doctor suggests. This may include breast cancer information, articles about breast cancer, and good websites. These can help you make decisions about your treatment.

Should I consider genetic testing?[6]

Experts agree that genetic testing should be considered only when there is a reasonable suspicion that a genetic mutation may be present.

Some inherited gene changes can greatly raise a woman's risk for breast cancer and may affect treatment decisions. Although women may have relatives with breast cancer, in most cases, their cancer is *not* because of an inherited gene mutation.

If you have relatives with breast cancer (or certain other cancers) or relatives who had breast cancer at a young age, talk with your doctor before you decide to seek counseling. Women with a strong family history of breast cancer may be referred to a genetic counselor who can talk with them about the risks and benefits of genetic testing. Widespread screening of the general public is not recommended.

Genetic tests look for mutations in the *BRCA1* and *BRCA2* genes, most commonly. Genetic counselors can also advise whether other members of the patient's family should consider testing.

What should I do if I have an inherited genetic mutation?[6]

Knowing about a genetic mutation can affect treatment decisions for women who already have breast cancer.

These decisions can include whether to choose mastectomy or breast-conserving surgery or whether to have risk-reduction surgery, like removing the ovaries, or having the healthy breast removed. Talk with your doctor about the risks, benefits, and limits of your treatment options.

How is surgery used to treat breast cancer?

Doctors perform surgery to cut the cancer away from healthy breast tissue.

Surgery is one of the most common treatments for breast cancer. The primary goal of breast cancer surgery is to remove the cancer from the breast and from the lymph nodes, if it has spread there. During surgery, the doctor may remove the cancer along with a small amount of breast tissue, or he or she may need to remove one or both of your breasts. These two kinds of breast cancer surgery are called lumpectomy and mastectomy.

- **Lumpectomy, or breast-conserving surgery,** is removing the lump, or tumor, and some of the breast tissue around it. If cancer is found at the edge of the tissue removed by surgery, the surgeon may need to remove more tissue. It's important to have clear, cancer-free margins of normal breast tissue to help prevent the cancer from coming back.

- **Mastectomy** is removing the full breast or both breasts. There are different types of mastectomies. For example, in a simple mastectomy just the breast is removed. In a modified radical mastectomy, the breast, the lining over the chest muscle, and some underarm lymph nodes are removed.

In many cases, breast-conserving surgeries combined with other treatments like radiation or chemotherapy can be as effective as modified radical mastectomy.

Lumpectomy/partial mastectomy

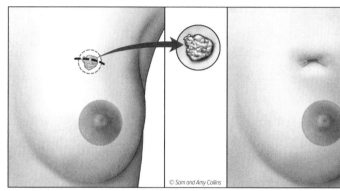

© Sam and Amy Collins

The tumor is removed with a rim of normal breast tissue.

Postoperative appearance depends on the amount of tissue removed, but there will be a small scar and often an indentation in the breast.

Modified radical mastectomy

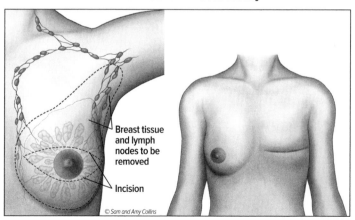

Breast tissue and lymph nodes to be removed

Incision

© Sam and Amy Collins

Postoperative appearance

What is the role of the lymph system in breast cancer?

Lymph nodes are small groups of immune cells in your body. They are connected by lymph vessels, which are like tiny blood vessels. Cancer cells can invade lymph vessels and spread to lymph nodes, where they can settle and grow. The lymph nodes in the underarm area near the breast are usually the first to be affected when breast cancer begins to spread. It is important that these lymph nodes are checked to see if the cancer has spread to them. If it has, it's a sign that the cancer may have spread to other organs.

The first lymph node that lymph fluid reaches after leaving the breast is called the sentinel node. This is the node that the cancer would be likely to spread to first.

In a sentinel lymph node biopsy (SLNB), the surgeon removes the node(s) for examination under a microscope. The SLNB can show whether cancer has spread to the lymph nodes without having to remove all of them.

If the sentinel node does not contain cancer, that usually means that no other lymph nodes need to be removed, because it's unlikely the cancer has reached them. But if the sentinel node does contain cancer, the underarm lymph nodes might need to be removed in a more extensive operation known as an axillary lymph node dissection (ALND).

The lymph system

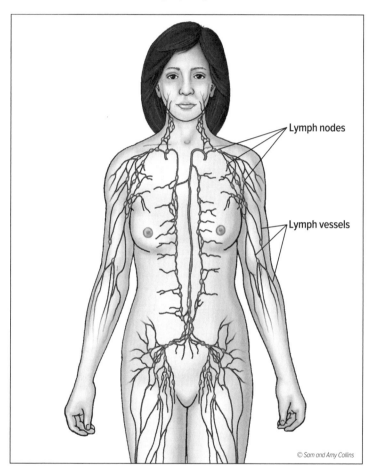

© Sam and Amy Collins

The lymph system has two main parts: lymph nodes and lymph vessels. Lymph nodes are connected by lymph vessels, which are like veins, except they carry lymph instead of blood.

Lymph nodes in relation to the breast

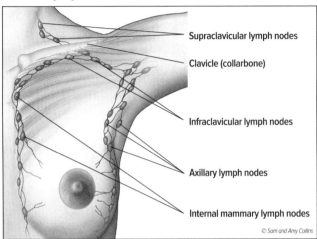

Supraclavicular lymph nodes

Clavicle (collarbone)

Infraclavicular lymph nodes

Axillary lymph nodes

Internal mammary lymph nodes

© Sam and Amy Collins

Sentinel lymph node biopsy

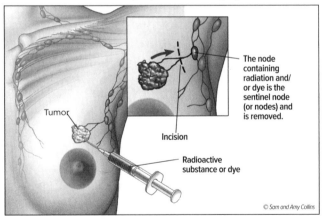

The node containing radiation and/ or dye is the sentinel node (or nodes) and is removed.

Tumor

Incision

Radioactive substance or dye

© Sam and Amy Collins

During a sentinel lymph node biopsy, a radioactive substance and/ or blue dye is injected into the tumor, near the tumor, or into the area around the nipple. That substance travels to the sentinel node, which is then removed to check for cancer.

An ALND might also be done if the lymph nodes are found to be enlarged during an exam or on an imaging test.

Axillary lymph node dissection

Lymph nodes removed

© Sam and Amy Collins

Postoperative appearance

How do I decide between mastectomy and lumpectomy?

Think about how each type of surgery might affect your life.

Read the following information about each procedure. Then, talk with your doctor about your choices.

? Questions ————————————

to think about when deciding which
type of surgery is best for you

1. What are the risks and benefits of having
    lumpectomy versus mastectomy?

2. How will I feel after losing one or both of my
    breasts?

3. Has my doctor recommended one approach over
    the other?

4. Am I at a high risk for cancer recurrence (cancer
    coming back)?

5. Would one type of surgery lower the chances of
    cancer recurring more than the other?

6. How many lymph nodes, if any, will need to be removed?

7. Will I need radiation therapy or other treatments after surgery? What is involved with radiation therapy? (See pages 55 and 56 to read more about radiation therapy.)

8. What side effects can I expect from the surgery? What can be done to help with these side effects? Which ones should be reported right away?

9. What if I decide to have breast reconstruction surgery after mastectomy? What will be involved? (See the following pages and pages 121–137 to read about options after a mastectomy.)

What Should I Expect After a Mastectomy?

A mastectomy usually takes 2 to 3 hours. Surgery will take longer if you are also having reconstructive surgery. After the surgery, you will probably stay in the hospital for 1 or 2 nights. When you wake up after surgery, you will see a bandage over your breast area. You also may have one or more drains (plastic or rubber tubes) in your breast or underarm area. These drains remove blood and lymph fluids that collect while you are healing. The drains will need to stay in place for 1 to 2 weeks.

You will need to see your doctor a week or two after surgery for follow-up and to have the drains removed.

Women are often surprised by how little pain they have in the breast area after surgery. However, there may be strange sensations, like a feeling of numbness, pinching, or pulling in the underarm area.

Talk with your doctor about how to take care of yourself after surgery. Your treatment may include radiation or chemotherapy. See information about these treatments on pages 55–58.

Before leaving the hospital, you should received printed instructions for how to care for yourself at home. The instructions should include all the issues listed on the next 2 pages.

What to ask ———
about caring for yourself
after mastectomy

How to take care of your body:

- How to take care of the surgical wound and bandage

- How to monitor and take care of the drains

- How to recognize the signs of infection

- How to bathe and shower after surgery

- What medicines to take (including pain medicines) and how often

- When to call your doctor or nurse

How to get back into your life:

- What foods you should eat or not eat

- What activities you should do or not do

- How soon you can return to work

continued on next page

continued from previous page

How to get used to your body after surgery:

- When to start using your arm

- How to exercise your arm to keep it from getting stiff

- When you will be able to wear a breast form. A breast form is padding shaped like a breast that can be worn under clothing.

- What to do about feelings you may have about how you look

- How to get in touch with an American Cancer Society Reach To Recovery® volunteer. Reach To Recovery is a program in which breast cancer patients can talk by phone, face-to-face, or electronically with other breast cancer survivors. See the resources guide on page 180 for more information about this program.

What Should I Expect After a Lumpectomy?

Breast-conserving surgery, or lumpectomy, usually takes less than 1 hour. Most of the time, a lumpectomy will be done on an outpatient basis, and this does not require an overnight stay in the hospital.

After a lumpectomy, you may have a drain (tube) coming out of your armpit. This is usually taken out before you leave the hospital. Sometimes the drain needs to stay in longer and may be removed at your follow-up visit with your doctor (about a week after surgery).

After your surgery, you may need radiation treatment. Radiation treatments are typically given 5 days a week (Monday through Friday) for about 5 weeks. However, a shorter duration of treatment (or another form of radiation) may be an option for some patients.[7-9] If you are getting chemotherapy, your doctor may want you to wait to get radiation therapy. See pages 55 and 56 for more information about radiation therapy after breast-conserving surgery.

Women are often surprised by how little pain they have in the breast area after surgery. But they may feel numbness, pinching, or pulling in the underarm area.

Most doctors want you to start moving your arm soon after surgery so it won't get stiff.

continued on next page

continued from previous page

Talk with your doctor about how to take care of yourself after surgery. Before leaving the hospital, you should receive a printed form with instructions for how to care for yourself at home. The instructions should include all the issues listed on the next 2 pages.

What to ask

about caring for yourself
after lumpectomy

How to take care of your body:

- How to take care of the wound and bandage

- How to take care of the drains

- How to know if you have an infection

- What medicines to take (including pain medicines) and how often

- When to call your doctor or nurse

How to get back into your life:

- What foods you should eat or not eat

- What activities you should do or not do

- How soon you can return to work

continued on next page

continued from previous page

How to get used to your body after surgery:

- When to start using your affected arm

- How to exercise your arm to keep it from getting stiff

- How to get in touch with an American Cancer Society Reach To Recovery® volunteer. Reach To Recovery is a program in which breast cancer patients can talk by phone, face-to-face, or electronically with other breast cancer survivors. See the resource guide on page 180 for more information about this program.

What are other treatments for breast cancer?

How is radiation therapy used to treat breast cancer?

Radiation therapy uses special x-rays to kill or harm cancer cells.

Radiation therapy may be used as the main treatment for a cancer, to reduce the size of a cancer before surgery, or to destroy any remaining cancer cells after surgery. It may also be used as a palliative treatment. Palliative care relieves cancer symptoms and helps with side effects of treatment.

There are 2 main ways radiation therapy is given:

- A special machine is used to point powerful x-rays at the cancer from outside the body. This is known as external radiation therapy. This type of treatment is like getting an x-ray and is painless, even though the radiation used is much stronger.

- Tiny pellets containing radiation are placed in the breast for a short time. This type of treatment, known as internal radiation therapy or brachytherapy, can be used after a lumpectomy. A long, thin device is placed in the space where the breast tumor was removed with one end sticking out of the breast. This device stays in place until treatment is complete. The radioactive pellets are typically placed in the device for a short time and removed twice each day over 5 days.

Radiation hurts cancer cells, but it also hurts healthy cells. The treatment can cause side effects like muscle stiffness, mild swelling and tenderness, and a sunburn-like reaction on the skin where you received radiation. These side effects should go away as the normal, healthy cells recover.

How is chemotherapy used to treat breast cancer?

Chemotherapy uses drugs to kill or harm cancer cells.[10]

Chemotherapy drugs stop cancer cells from growing and dividing. Chemotherapy may be used before or after surgery to destroy any cancer cells still in your body. It can also be used to help shrink or slow the growth of advanced breast cancers.

Chemotherapy is given in cycles, with treatment days followed by days of rest to help the body recover. The length of the chemotherapy cycle varies by the specific drug or combination of drugs.

There are 2 main ways chemotherapy is given:

- "Chemo" drugs are given intravenously (IV, or into a vein). The drugs travel through the body in the bloodstream.

- Chemotherapy can also be given in pill form.

Like radiation therapy, chemotherapy can also cause damage to healthy cells. This can result in side effects like nausea, vomiting, fatigue, mouth sores, hair loss, and low blood cell counts. These side effects should go away as the normal, healthy cells recover. See pages 68–88 for more information about side effects.

A woman having chemotherapy for breast cancer usually takes 2 or more different chemotherapy drugs for 3 to 6 months. However, the length of treatment also depends on why chemo is being given, how well it is working, and what side effects occur.

How is hormone therapy used to treat breast cancer?

Hormone therapy uses drugs to change the way hormones work in the body. It helps stop cancer cells from growing.[11]

Hormones are chemicals made in the body. Certain kinds of breast cancer need hormones so they can grow. If the hormones are blocked, cancer cells can't grow.

Hormone therapy is used most often after surgery to lower the chances of cancer coming back. It can also be used to treat breast cancer that has come back or spread to other parts of your body. Sometimes it is used with chemotherapy.

Not all types of breast cancer can be treated with hormone therapy. Women with breast tumors that are estrogen receptor–positive (ER+) and/or progesterone receptor–positive (PR+) are likely to benefit from hormone therapy. These types of tumors represent about 2 out of 3 breast cancers. Based on the tests done on your breast cancer tissue, your doctor will know if you have the type of breast cancer that will be likely to respond to this kind of treatment.

How is targeted therapy used to treat breast cancer?

Targeted therapy helps the body fight cancer cells.[12]

Targeted drugs work differently from standard chemotherapy drugs. They attack certain parts of cancer cells that normally help the cells grow.

For example, about 1 in 5 breast cancers has too much of the growth-promoting protein HER2 on the surface of the cancer cells. HER2-positive breast cancers tend to grow and spread more quickly. Some drugs that target HER2 can help treat these cancers.

Side effects from targeted drugs are often different from those with chemotherapy and may be less severe.

For breast cancer, targeted therapy is most often used along with chemotherapy. From the tests done on your breast cancer tissue, your doctor will know whether you have the type of breast cancer that will be likely to respond to this type of treatment.

How is bone-directed therapy used to treat breast cancer?

Bone-directed therapy uses certain drugs to slow the growth of cancer in the bones. It may even prevent breast cancer from spreading to the bones in the first place.[13]

Drugs such as bisphosphonates and RANKL inhibitors can help strengthen the bones. Bone-directed therapy can lower the risk of fractures in bones weakened by breast cancer that has spread. These drugs are injected into a vein or under the skin.

Most doctors recommend that women have a dental checkup and have any tooth problems treated before taking these drugs. Maintaining good oral hygiene by flossing, brushing, and making sure that any dentures fit properly can help prevent a rare, but serious side effect of damage in the jaw bones.

What should I know about herbs, dietary supplements, or special diets to treat breast cancer?[14]

These treatments don't cure cancer.

When you have cancer, you may want to believe that there is a simple, easy way to fix it. But when something sounds too good to be true, it usually is. There isn't an herb, supplement, or diet that has been shown to cure breast cancer. Some might be helpful in certain ways (like helping relieve some side effects from treatment), but others might not help, or might even affect your other treatments. If you are thinking about adding an herb, supplement, or special diet to your cancer treatment, please talk with your doctor first. Find out about how the vitamins, herbs, or other therapies might affect your cancer treatment and whether they cause side effects.

Your doctor needs to know about any supplement or medicine you take. You may also consult with your pharmacist about supplements and whether they can interfere with your regular treatment.

Making Your Treatment Choices

Your doctor has probably given you a lot of information about treatment. You may feel overwhelmed by your treatment choices. In fact, some women prefer to have their doctors make their treatment decisions. Other women want to learn all they can and then make their own choices. Whatever you decide is okay.

If you want to be involved in your treatment decisions, here are some questions to ask:

- How effective is this treatment for my breast cancer?
- What will happen to me during treatment and how will it affect my life?
- What are the possible side effects from this treatment?
- Is there someone I could talk to who has been through the same treatment?

No one expects you to become an expert on cancer treatment. But you may feel more in control if you understand your choices and what may happen.

The American Cancer Society's Reach To Recovery volunteers can talk with you about cancer treatments and also share their own experiences with you. Call **800-227-2345** for more information about this program.

What Is a Clinical Trial?

It is a type of research study.

Clinical trials test medicines and/or procedures to see if they are safe and effective for people with cancer (or other diseases).

Thousands of people take part in clinical trials each year. Your doctor may want you to think about being part of a clinical trial. Ask your doctor why he or she thinks it might help you and what you can expect to happen during the study.

A person must be matched with a clinical trial. For example, to be part of a breast cancer clinical trial, a woman may need to meet requirements such as these:

- Have a certain type, stage, and grade of cancer
- Be within a certain age range
- Have not yet received treatment
- Have already received a certain treatment

There are benefits and risks to being in a clinical trial. You may be able to get a promising new treatment that is not yet available to the public. By taking part in a clinical trial, you may also help other people by making it possible for doctors to learn more about how to treat your type of breast cancer. On the other hand, no one can be sure how a new treatment will work, which is what the study is meant to find out. Some people might not be helped by the new treatment, or might even be harmed.

Here are some important points to consider before taking part in a clinical trial:

- You might not get to choose the treatment you get.
- You may need to travel often to the clinic for additional tests.
- Your treatment may cause side effects that doctors don't yet know about.

Remember:

- Taking part in a clinical trial is your choice. No one can force you to take part. You also have the right to drop out of a clinical trial if you decide it's not right for you.
- The Affordable Care Act requires that newer health insurance plans cover the routine costs of care for people who are in approved clinical trials.

For more information about clinical trials, call the American Cancer Society at **800-227-2345**, or visit our website at **cancer.org** and search for "clinical trials matching service."

Questions
to ask the doctor about treatments

1. Which treatment(s) do you think would work best for my cancer?

2. Will the treatment(s) get rid of all the cancer or help me live longer?

3. Will the treatment(s) make my life better? If so, how?

4. How well does the treatment usually work on my type and stage of breast cancer?

5. Are there other treatments we can try if this one doesn't get rid of my cancer? If so, which ones?

6. When would the treatment(s) happen and for how long?

7. Would I need to stay in the hospital for treatment? If so, for how long?

8. What steps would I need to take to get ready for treatment?

9. How soon do I need to start treatment?

10. What are the possible risks or problems of this treatment?

11. How will you know if the treatment is working?

12. When do I need to make my treatment decision?

Side Effects of Chemotherapy

Common Side Effects

- feeling sick to your stomach
- not feeling hungry
- bowel irregularity
- a change in the foods you like
- hair loss
- feeling tired
- irritation or sores in the mouth
- easy bruising or bleeding
- a greater chance of infections
- irritability
- trouble thinking or remembering

Less Common/Rare Side Effects

- damage to your heart, liver, or kidneys
- hearing loss
- nerve damage in your hands, feet, and/or legs
- getting a second cancer later in life
- nail changes (like a change in color)

What do I need to know about side effects from treatment?

What are side effects?

Side effects are unwanted symptoms or problems that happen because of treatment.[15]

Most cancer treatments cause side effects. Here's why. These treatments are strong enough to kill your cancer cells, but they can also harm the healthy cells in your body. As your healthy cells are harmed, you may feel sick, tired, or experience hair loss. Most of these side effects go away after your treatment is over.

There are ways to help prevent or stop some side effects. Ask your doctor about these issues:

- The possible side effects of the treatment
- How likely it is you will have side effects
- What can be done to prevent the side effects or deal with them if you get them
- How long the side effects are likely to last
- If the side effects will go away after your treatment is done

Will treatment make me feel sick?

Cancer treatment can make you feel sick to your stomach. It also can change your taste or desire for food.

What happens:

A few minutes or hours after you have chemotherapy, you might feel sick to your stomach or throw up. Sometimes other types of treatments might also make you feel sick. You may find that you don't feel much like eating, or that certain foods smell or taste different. These are common side effects and should go away after your treatment ends. Your doctor may be able to help with these side effects.

What you can do:

Ask your doctor about medicines you can take to help you feel better. You also may want to try the tips below.

What to eat:

- Eat foods without much taste or smell, like dry toast and crackers.
- Try Popsicles or Jell-O.
- Slowly sip cold, clear drinks like ginger ale.
- Eat foods with smells you like, and try lemon drops or mints.

How to eat:

- Eat small meals throughout the day.
- Eat food cold or at room temperature. It has less smell and taste than hot food.
- Try to rest for an hour after you eat a meal.
- Try to relax and take slow, deep breaths when you feel sick.

Will I lose my hair?

Some cancer treatments may make you lose your hair initially, but it almost always grows back.

What happens:

Many women lose their hair after a few weeks of chemotherapy, and some lose it during other drug treatments. Other women have problems with thinning hair, but don't lose all their hair. Some women lose hair from their eyebrows, eyelashes, and from other parts of their body. How much hair you lose depends on which medicines you take, how much of them you take, and how long you take them.

Many women worry about losing their hair. This is normal. Not many people are comfortable with hair loss. Our hair has a lot to do with how we feel about ourselves.

If you lose your hair, it will almost always start to grow back after your treatment ends. Sometimes when hair grows back, it is a different color or has a different texture.

What you can do:

Here are some ideas to help you cope with hair loss:

- Think about cutting your hair short before it starts to fall out (usually within a week or so of starting treatment).

- Call your health insurance company to find out whether they will pay for a wig. Then ask your doctor for a prescription for a wig.

- Choose a wig before treatment starts or early in your treatment if you want to match your hair color and texture.

- Ask your doctor or nurse for a list of wig shops, or look in the phone book. The American Cancer Society's "*tlc*" catalog has a wide selection of hats and wigs. Call **800-850-9445** to request a catalog.

- Wear a pretty hat, turban, or scarf instead of a wig.

- Wear sunscreen to protect your bare scalp, and wear a hat in cold weather and at night to keep in body heat.

- Attend a Look Good Feel Better® program, which is a free program that teaches beauty techniques to female cancer patients to help manage appearance–related side effects. To find a program in your area, call **800-227-2345**.

Will I feel tired?

Some people feel really tired during and after cancer treatment.

What happens:

The most common side effect of cancer treatment is fatigue. Fatigue is different from the tired feeling you get when you haven't had enough sleep. It is more like your brain, body, and emotions are all tired.

Fatigue can occur during chemotherapy or after a few weeks of radiation therapy. Fatigue will usually go away within a few months after treatment.

What you can do:

If you feel really tired, try the following steps:

- Take care of yourself.
- Get enough sleep.
- Eat well.
- Ask your doctor about drugs that might help.
- Exercise if you can—it may give you more energy.

Set limits:

- Don't force yourself do more than you feel you can.
- Decide which things are most important for you to do. Get a lot of rest and save your energy for those things.
- Let other people help you. Ask for help when you need it.

What is lymphedema? Will I get it?

Lymphedema appears as swelling of the arm. It can start after some treatments that affect the lymph nodes in your underarm.

Most women who have had breast cancer won't have this side effect.

What happens:

Lymphedema is a buildup of fluid that causes the arm to swell. It can occur after surgery or radiation therapy that affects the underarm area. The amount of swelling varies for each woman. Some women may have swelling that makes their rings feel tight on their fingers. For other women, it can make their arm swell to twice its normal size.

The chance of getting lymphedema varies a great deal, depending on the type of surgery a woman has and whether she gets radiation therapy. For example, the risk of lymphedema after lumpectomy alone is very low, whereas the risk after a modified radical mastectomy followed by radiation to the underarm area is much higher.[16,17]

The risk for lymphedema also goes up with these factors:

- Greater number of lymph nodes removed
- Being overweight or obese

How to lower your chances of getting lymphedema[18]:

- **Try to avoid infection and injury to the arm.** Keep the skin clean and protect it when you have cuts, scratches, or burns. Always wear gloves when gardening or doing dishes. Have blood drawn and have shots and other medical procedures done on the other arm, if possible.

- **Try to avoid burns.** Protect your arm from sunburn. Use oven mitts when cooking. Avoid splash burns from microwaved and steaming foods. Avoid hot tubs and saunas. The heat can cause fluid buildup.

- **Try to avoid clothing or other items that squeeze or put pressure on the affected arm or shoulder.** Avoid using shoulder straps when carrying briefcases and purses. Have your blood pressure taken on the other arm (or on the thigh when both arms are affected).

- **Ask about a specially fitted sleeve.** If you have lymphedema or there is concern about developing it, talk with your doctor or physical therapist about whether you would benefit from wearing a specially fitted sleeve over your arm. If recommended, you may need to get a prescription from your doctor so your insurance will cover the cost.

- **Try to keep your arm elevated when you can.** For example, when you are seated, rest your arm on the back of a sofa or armrest. Gravity from having your arms down at your sides all day can promote fluid buildup.

- **Try to avoid muscle strain.** It's okay to do your normal activities with the affected arm, but don't overdo it. Exercise, but try not to overtire your arm. Talk with your doctor about the level of activity that is right for you. If you have to carry heavy items, use your unaffected arm, or both arms.

Watch for signs of lymphedema if multiple lymph nodes were removed during your surgery, or if you've had radiation therapy to the underarm area. Look at your upper body in front of a mirror every 2 weeks. Call your doctor if you notice any of these signs:

- A full or tight feeling in your arm
- The arm on the side of the body where your cancer was treated looks bigger than the other
- Weakness in your arm or not being able to move it as far as before
- Skin changes, like skin that stays pushed in after you press on it

Call the American Cancer Society at **800-227-2345** for more information about how to take care of your arm and lower your chances of having lymphedema.

Could I have other side effects?

Yes. Ask your doctor about other possible side effects.

Other possible side effects of cancer treatment include—

- **"Chemo brain."** Chemotherapy can result in memory issues; that is, after treatments you may have a hard time thinking or remembering things. This problem is often referred to as "chemo brain."

- **Mouth sores.** Mouth sores can be another unpleasant and painful side effect from cancer treatments and can interfere with eating.

- **Skin and breast changes.** Radiation therapy can turn your skin red like a sunburn, make your skin feel thicker, or change the size of your breast. These changes usually go away 6 to 12 months after treatment. Chemotherapy can also make your skin itchy and dry or cause it to peel.

- **Getting sick more easily.** Some treatments can weaken your body so that you get sick, bleed, or bruise more easily than before.

- **Hot flashes, vaginal discharge, and other effects of hormone therapy.** Other side effects may include vaginal dryness and/or itching, irregular menstrual periods, headache, nausea, skin rash, fatigue, and weight gain.

- **Changes in bowel habits.** You might be constipated or have diarrhea during chemotherapy.

- **More chance of getting another cancer.** It is very rare, but sometimes treatment can make another cancer grow in your body. If this should happen, it would be years after your breast cancer treatment.

Is there help for any pain I might have?

Yes. Doctors can help you feel better if you are in pain.

Tell your doctor about any pain you feel. Pain can be a sign that something is wrong in your body. Tell your doctor when the pain started, how long it lasts, and if anything makes it better or worse. Also, tell the doctor how bad your pain is on a scale of 1 to 10, with 1 as the lowest amount of pain and 10 as the very worst pain. And follow these steps:

- **Take your pain medicine when the doctor tells you to.** Don't wait until the pain is really bad to take your medicine. It is easier to stop pain before it starts or keep pain under control than to get rid of serious pain once it starts.

- **Tell your doctor about any side effects from the medicine.** Pain medicines may make you feel sick or constipated, but other medicines or laxatives can help with these problems.

- **Don't stop taking your pain medicine all at once.** Ask your doctor before stopping. He or she may have you taper the doses. That is, take a little less each day until you are off the medicine.

There are many types of pain medicine. If one pain reliever doesn't work for you, talk with your doctor about trying another. You should get enough pain relief to be able to do the things that are important to you.

Can I cope with side effects like pain without medicine?

There are many ways you can feel better without taking medicine.[14]

The methods below may help you deal with side effects or just feel better. You can get information on these and other ways of helping your mind and body from some hospitals and health centers. The staff there can train you in these techniques or help you find professionals who do them. Or you may be able to find classes at gyms and community centers.

- **Acupuncture** may help with nausea from chemotherapy,[19] but talk to your doctor before you start.[20] A professional acupuncturist inserts very thin needles into specific points on the skin.

- **Aromatherapy** may help with mood, anxiety, and stress. Essential oils (fragrant substances from plants) are either inhaled or massaged into the body.

- **Hypnosis** may help with pain, fear, anxiety, and hot flashes.[21] Hypnosis is one way of putting people in a state of relaxation, but with focus on a certain problem or side effect.

- **Imagery** may help with nausea and vomiting from chemotherapy, relieve stress, and help with weight gain, depression, and pain. It involves doing mental exercises, like thinking of a goal and imagining reaching it.

- **Massage** may help lower stress and anxiety. It also may help with fatigue and pain. It involves rubbing and kneading muscles, which helps you relax.[22]

- **Meditation** may help with pain, anxiety, and high blood pressure. It is a way of concentrating that relaxes your body and calms your mind. It can create a sense of well-being.

- **Relaxation** can relieve pain, help you fall asleep, give you more energy, make you feel less tired, lower your anxiety, and make other pain relief methods work better. There are different relaxation methods, like thinking of a peaceful, calm scene or breathing slowly and focusing on your breathing.

- **Spirituality** can help by lowering your stress and anxiety and helping you have a more positive outlook. It is an awareness of something greater than one's self and usually involves religion and prayer.

- **Tai chi** can help lower your stress, heart rate, and blood pressure levels. Tai chi is an exercise that involves movement, meditation, and breathing. It may help with posture, balance, flexibility, and strength.

- **Yoga** can help relieve some symptoms of cancer. Yoga is a type of exercise that involves different postures and breathing. It can help you relax and get physically fit.

Remember, there is no one "right" way to treat your pain. It's okay to try medicine along with some of the methods listed above for pain relief and other side effects. You need to find out what works for you.

Will I be able to have children after treatment?

It depends on the type of cancer treatment you get.

If you think you may want to have children in the future, talk with your doctor about it before you begin your treatment. Some chemotherapy drugs can make you unable to have children for a while or forever. Other medicines, like hormone therapy, might not be safe to take if you get pregnant.

Any problems you have getting pregnant after treatment will depend mainly on these factors:

- How old you are during treatment
- How much chemotherapy you have and for how long
- Which chemotherapy drugs you take

Ask if there is anything you can do before treatment starts that could help your chances of having children after treatment ends.

Questions
to ask the doctor about
side effects

1. What are the possible side effects of this treatment?

2. How long might side effects last?

3. Will I feel tired or sick during treatment?

4. Will any of the side effects change how I look, either for a short time or for good?

5. Could another treatment fight my cancer but affect my life in a different way?

6. Which side effects should I expect right away?

continued on next page

continued from previous page

7. Which side effects should I expect later?

8. What side effects should I call you about right away?

9. Can anything be done to stop, or lessen, side effects before they start?

10. How should I take care of my skin, breast, or body during treatment?

11. Are there any services or programs that can help me cope with side effects?

What should I know about paying for treatment?

How can I get help to pay for my treatment?

You may be able to get help paying for your health care.[23]

The Affordable Care Act has an open enrollment period each year. During this time, people who don't have health insurance through their jobs and are not currently receiving Medicare can shop for a health plan on their state's marketplace. The health care law ensures that all health plans sold in the health insurance marketplaces cover essential benefits such as cancer screening, treatment, and follow-up care.

The American Cancer Society Health Insurance Assistance Service (HIAS) educates cancer patients, cancer survivors, individuals with cancer symptoms, and those calling on their behalf about health insurance options available during the Affordable Care Act open enrollment. Patients and their advocates should call **800-227-2345** and ask to speak with someone from HIAS for questions about health insurance plans to fit their needs.

The American Cancer Society can provide other information about private health insurance plans, government programs like Medicare, and other sources of financial help. See the resource guide on pages 175–183.

What do Medicare and Medicaid pay for?

These government programs may pay for some of your medical care, but not all of it.

You must first qualify for Medicare or Medicaid before they will pay for any of your medical care. You may be able to get Medicare if you are 65 years or older or if you get Social Security benefits because you are disabled. You may be able to get Medicaid if you make less than a certain amount of money or are disabled.

It can be confusing to figure out what medical costs are covered by these programs. Call Medicare at **800-633-4227** or visit their website at **medicare.gov** to find out which cancer treatments and medicines are covered. You also can ask a social worker or case manager at your hospital about Medicare, or call the American Cancer Society at **800-227-2345** with questions.

Are there other groups that can help me pay for my treatment and other costs?

There are private groups that may help you pay for your treatment and other living costs.

Talk with the social worker at your hospital. Also, see the resource guide on pages 175–183, or call the American Cancer Society at **800-227-2345** for information on how to get help from these organizations:

- **Community groups** like the Salvation Army, Catholic Social Services, United Way, Jewish Social Services, and others

- **National groups** such as CancerCare that offer help and information about paying for expenses and other practical help

What if I can't pay my bills?[24]

Explain what is happening. Ask for more time or other help.

Many people have a hard time paying bills at one time or another. It is nothing to be ashamed of. Most hospitals and other companies will listen to your story and try to help. Try taking the steps below:

- Ask to pay the bill later or in a few payments instead of one.
- Explain the problem to hospital billing staff. Ask about payment options.
- Talk with a social worker at the hospital about ways you can get help for a while with money challenges.
- Think about letting relatives or friends help out with money for a while. If they know what you're going through, they may want to help. It may be hard to accept this type of help. But by helping you, your friends and family may feel they are helping you get through cancer treatment.

What is private health insurance? What does it pay for?

Private health insurance is insurance you get through work or that you pay for on your own. These plans may pay for many treatment costs.

The medical care, drugs, and supplies that health insurance pays for are called benefits. If you have health insurance, look at the terms of your policy and make notes about what expenses are covered and which ones are not covered. Insurance may not pay for prescription drugs, counseling, or care in your home. Some insurance plans have programs that include nurses or case managers to help you manage your care. Check your policy to see if you have this type of benefit. Ask if you can get more insurance benefits through a catastrophic illness clause.

What if my insurance claim is turned down?

Ask for help. The insurance company may still cover your claim.

The bills sent to the insurance company by you or your doctor are called claims. Keep track of your bills and send claims to your health insurance company as soon as you get them. Hospitals, clinics, and doctors' offices usually have someone who can help you fill out claim forms.

Sometimes an insurance company won't pay one of your bills. If this happens, ask your doctor's office or the hospital claims office for help. They may be able to look at the claim form and find the problem. Also, call your insurance company and find out how to appeal a claim that has been turned down. This means that you submit the claim again and ask the company to pay.

Keep copies of important papers: claims, letters of medical necessity, bills, explanation of benefits, receipts, requests for sick leave from work, and any letters to and from the insurance company. These records will help you get payment for your medical bills.

? Questions

to ask the hospital billing department or insurance company

1. How much will my cancer treatment cost?

2. Will I get separate bills from the hospital, surgeon, and other doctors?

3. Is this treatment covered by most insurance plans?

4. How much of the costs will my insurance cover?

5. If I don't have insurance or the treatment isn't covered by my insurance, are there any ways I can get help paying for it?

What Is a Breast Cancer Survivor?

Many women choose to think of themselves as breast cancer survivors. Survivor is a word some people use to mean anyone who has received a cancer diagnosis. Someone living with breast cancer could therefore be called a breast cancer survivor. Other people use the word survivor to mean someone who has finished cancer treatment or who has lived several years after a diagnosis of cancer.

Not everyone thinks of herself as a survivor. Some people would rather not be called a survivor. This is a personal choice.

How will cancer and treatment affect me and my loved ones?

Does anyone feel the way I do?

Yes, others may feel the way you do.

Some women feel confused and upset about having breast cancer.[25] It's normal to be worried, sad, or angry.

Here's how some women with breast cancer feel:

- "I feel like I will be a burden to my family if I take time to go to doctors, if I'm not feeling well, or if we have to pay for treatment."

- "I worry about my family and how upset they will be more than I worry about myself."

- "I worry about how to talk to my children about my breast cancer."

- "I worry that my partner will leave me or that future partners won't think I'm pretty because I have cancer or I've had a breast removed."

- "I'm afraid of what will happen in my life and what will happen to my body."

You might have some of these same worries. Don't be tough on yourself. It is hard to adjust to having cancer and getting treatment. It affects so many parts of your life. You are bound to worry sometimes. You will feel better on some days than others.

If you feel really down and find yourself thinking about death or harming yourself, you may have signs of clinical depression. This is very serious. Tell your doctor right away if you have any thoughts or feelings like this.

How can I feel more in control of my life?

Think about ways you can deal with your fears or challenges.

It might help to think through what worries you, then think of ways you can deal with each of your fears or challenges. For example, if you're worried about how you would look without your breast, talk with women who have had mastectomies. Ask them about their experiences. Find out what they did to cope.

You may be worried that the cancer will come back. This is a common fear among breast cancer survivors.[26] Such fears may get stronger after treatment ends, when you are no longer seeing your health care team for regular treatment and feeling their support. If you still have feelings of uncertainty about your health and the future, this may impact your quality of life.[27] Talk with your doctor about finding help for anxiety, whether it's joining a support group, seeing a counselor, or starting new activities to stay healthy and keep your mind focused on things other than your health. (See other suggestions on the following pages.)

Your concerns may be related to everyday tasks, which may seem less important. Maybe you're worried that vacuuming will hurt your arm and that you won't be able to do it. You could ask a friend to help you with chores, or you could trade less active chores with a friend or neighbor. Any worry you have is perfectly okay—every woman is different, and no concern is silly.

Think of the things that worry you—whatever they are—and write them down. Then write down as many ideas as you can that may help you feel more in control. Think about who can help you.

Start with your biggest worries:

1. **I'm afraid or worried that . . .**
   What are all the ways I can think of to make this better?

2. **I'm afraid or worried that . . .**
   What are all the ways I can think of to make this better?

3. **I'm afraid or worried that . . .**
   What are all the ways I can think of to make this better?

Keeping a Journal May Help

Think about keeping a journal. It's a helpful way to get out feelings like anger, confusion, fear, or guilt.

Write down what happens in your life. Describe what it feels like to have cancer. Write about how other people react to the news that you have cancer. Write about what happens when you see the doctor or how you feel about your treatment choices. You can also use your journal to record and track medical tests and procedures so you will know what to expect if you have them again.

Writing about your feelings may help you cope with your cancer and feel better. You may want to begin writing in your journal by finishing these sentences.

1. When I first found out I had cancer, I felt . . .

2. I wish that I . . .

3. I can make this happen by doing . . .

4. One of the things I worry about most is . . .

5. What would make me feel better is . . .

6. When I tell other people about my cancer . . .

7. I feel closest to other people when . . .

8. I get upset when . . .

9. When I get mad I . . .

10. When things get to be too much I . . .

11. I would like to deal with things by . . .

12. I couldn't get through this without . . .

13. The best times I have are . . .

14. What I like most about myself is . . .

How can I find help and support?

There are many places that can help you.

Going to support groups with other women who have breast cancer can be a way for you to—

- talk about your feelings, your fears, and the changes in your life;
- hear what has happened to other women and learn from them;
- spend time with women who understand what you're going through;
- help other women and let them help you; and
- learn about other kinds of help in your area.

Talk with your doctor or call the American Cancer Society at **800-227-2345** to find out about support groups in your area.

You also can check pages 175–183 in the resource guide for more information about support groups.

I told my family that I have breast cancer. Why are they acting strangely?

Family members may act strangely because they are afraid.

Family members may not know how to act. Their fears probably are related to—

- worries about losing you;
- what will happen to them if something happens to you;
- not knowing how to help you;
- worrying about not being strong enough when you need them; and
- worries about the cancer itself.

You may be able to help your family by opening up to them. Talk about what you think will happen, how you feel, and how treatment may affect you. If you want, tell them they can ask you questions and talk with you about your cancer. This may help all of you feel more comfortable. If you need help talking with your children about your cancer, please call the American Cancer Society at **800-227-2345**.[28]

How will cancer affect my friendships?

Friends will react to your news in different ways.

Some friends will offer help right away or try to make you feel better. Others may stay away from you because they don't know what to say or do. They may be afraid of what may happen to you. Or they may worry that they might say the wrong thing. Some may even think they can catch cancer from you. (This can't happen. People don't get cancer from other people.) Some friends may be upset if you don't feel well enough to spend time with them or go to get-togethers.

It is natural for friends to want things to be like they used to be, before you had cancer. Read the next section to find out how to talk with your friends about your cancer.

How can I talk to family and friends about cancer?

Try to be honest and let them know what's happening.[29]

If it feels okay, tell friends and family members these facts:

- That you have breast cancer (they may feel hurt if they hear the news from someone else)

- That you expect to use your strength and many resources to get through treatment

- That you can't give them cancer

Let them ask questions and tell them what you've learned about breast cancer. If someone says something that hurts your feelings, let that person know. But try to understand if people seem to act funny or distant. Like you, they're figuring out what to say and how they feel.

If you aren't comfortable talking about personal things, it's okay not to open up about your feelings or your cancer. This is one place where you are in control.

How will cancer treatment affect my life at home?

You may not be able to do everything you used to do.

Your daily life may need to change because of your cancer treatment. You may feel tired or sick and just not have much energy. This means that you'll need to do less at home and others will need to do more. Talk with your family members and friends about how they can help.

Give them something specific to do. Ask them to pick up the kids from school, do the dishes, bring over a meal, or run to the drugstore. Let them know that you'd like to talk about things other than cancer for a while. Or ask them just to sit and relax with you. People can help more when they know what really makes you feel better.

Can anyone help me with day-to-day challenges?

Special programs and trained staff may be able to help.

Some hospitals have staff who are trained to help you find programs that you may need. Your doctors, nurses, or social workers may be able to help you with the following:

- getting to and from your treatment;
- finding child care;
- getting help paying bills and solving insurance problems; and
- finding other resources in your community that can provide the support you need.

The American Cancer Society can help you find resources in your community. Our staff are trained to listen to you, learn your needs, and put together an action plan just for you. Call the American Cancer Society at **800-227-2345** for more information.

? Questions ———————

to ask the doctor, nurse, or social
worker about life during treatment

1. How will treatment affect my day-to-day life?

2. Will I need someone to drive me to and from
    treatment?

3. What changes should I expect at home during
    treatment? For example, will I need help with
    chores, have to cut back on my hobbies, or make
    other changes to my daily life?

4. How should I take care of my breast, skin, or
    surgery scar?

5. What else should I know about taking care of
    myself during treatment?

6. Will I have energy during treatment?

7. Will I be able to exercise?

8. Will I be able to travel out of town during treatment?

How will cancer and treatment affect my work?

Is it better to work during treatment or take time off?

If you have a choice and feel well enough, you may choose to continue working.[24,30]

Talk with your doctor about how your cancer treatment might affect your work. Ask whether you should take time off from your job, and how long you might need.

Many women want to feel as normal as possible during treatment. They choose to go back to work as soon as they can. Some women who have a lumpectomy (breast-conserving surgery) for early-stage breast cancer don't have side effects that stop them from going back to work. They sometimes go back to work a few days after surgery and work during radiation treatment. Other women take time off to let their bodies and minds rest. Not everyone feels ready to work during treatment or so soon after surgery. Only you and your doctor can decide what you are ready for.

Remember, there is no right or wrong choice about whether or not to work during your treatment. Whatever you decide is okay.

Should I tell people at work that I have cancer?

You may want to tell your coworkers if you will be taking time off.

It's up to you to decide how much to tell your coworkers about your breast cancer. They may be helpful and understanding, or they may feel uneasy and not know what to say or do.

If you think telling people at work will be a problem, first talk with a social worker at the hospital. He or she may be able to help you decide how much information you should share.

Could I lose my job if I have to take time off?

If you need to take time off, there are ways to protect your job.

You may choose not to tell your employer that you have cancer. Employers don't have a legal right to ask for information about your diagnosis or condition. If you expect to be away from the office for treatment, you will be required to obtain a doctor's note, indicating that you will be under the doctor's care for a certain amount of time. The note may include job-related limitations or restrictions, as well as an acknowledgment that you will need to take a leave of absence.

If you decide you can continue to work, think about telling your employer why you will need to take time off for treatments. Talk with your boss about how much time you expect to take off.

It's a good idea to keep track of all communications with your boss or with people in the benefits office. If you think you have been treated unfairly at work, call the U.S. Equal Employment Opportunity Commission (**800-669-4000**).

There are Federal laws that may protect your rights and your job while you are in treatment:

- **The Americans with Disabilities Act (ADA)** makes it illegal for an employer to punish you for having a disability like cancer. The ADA also may protect you if you are looking for a new job. To learn more, call **800-514-0301** or visit the ADA website at **ada.gov.**

- **The Family and Medical Leave Act (FMLA)** says that employers with 50 or more workers have to give workers up to 3 months of unpaid time off to take care of themselves or a family member. To qualify, you must have worked at least 1 year and worked at least 1,250 hours during that time. For more information, call the Wage and Hour Division of the U.S. Department of Labor at **866-4-USWAGE (866-487-9243)** or visit their website at **dol.gov/whd.**

How can I get ready to take time off from work?

A little planning will help you and your coworkers.

Before you take time off, consider discussing these options with your boss:

- Working different hours, working part time, or working from home
- Sharing work with other people
- Passing work on to others
- Making detailed lists of your projects and what needs to be done
- Telling people the status of your projects

Any of these options may make it easier for you to take time off from work, as well as make it easier for your boss and coworkers.

Can I get help with money if I'm not able to work?

You may have options for help.

Social workers or case managers at your hospital or organizations like the American Cancer Society can usually tell you about government or other programs that could help. Patient advocates or financial aid counselors at the hospital also may provide options. You may not think of yourself as disabled, but the programs below also help people being treated for cancer:

- **Long-term disability insurance:** If you can't work, find out if you have a long-term disability insurance policy through your job. This type of insurance may provide 60 to 70 percent of your income.

- **Social Security Disability Income (SSDI):** If you have been working for many years, SSDI may help you. Contact the Social Security Administration at **800-772-1213** or **ssa.gov** to find out how to apply. If you get turned down the first time, you can reapply. Any benefits won't begin until you have been disabled for 6 months.

- **Supplemental Security Income (SSI):** If you have not worked much or if you haven't earned very much, SSI may help you. You must be disabled, over 65 years old, and/or blind or visually impaired. Ask the social worker at the hospital or your local Social Security Administration office how to apply.

? Questions

to ask the social worker or doctor about work

1. Will I need to take time off from work?

2. If I need to stay home after treatment, how long will I be away from my job?

3. If I do go back to work, will I need a different work schedule?

4. Will I have a hard time doing any part of my job after treatment?

5. How will I know if I am overdoing it at my job?

6. Do I need to give my employer special forms before taking time off from work?

Recovering from Treatment

What if my breast was removed?

Will I ever get used to the changes in my body?

It takes time, but most women do adjust to these changes.

Cancer and treatment can change the way you feel about your body and yourself. This is normal. You have been through a serious illness and your body is different. After a while, most women do get used to their new bodies. They realize that women are beautiful and feminine whether they have two breasts, one breast, or none. But this takes time.

Most women are able to accept these changes within 1 or 2 years of treatment. For some women it takes longer. Each woman is different.

Give yourself time, and try the following steps:

- **Be patient.** If you have trouble looking at or touching your scars right away, don't worry. You may need to try many times to feel okay with the change.

- **Try to feel good about your whole body.** Just because one part of your body has changed does not mean you are ugly or less of a woman.

- **Don't be hard on yourself.** You don't have to feel happy about the changes. Don't feel like you have to fake it.

- **Join a support group.** Ask your doctor or a social worker at the hospital about support groups for women who have had mastectomies. Talking with other women who have been through the same thing can be really helpful and comforting.

What are my choices after a mastectomy?

You will likely have some choices after a mastectomy:

- **Doing nothing** to recreate your breast(s).

- **Wearing a prosthesis** or "breast form," which is shaped like a breast or part of a breast. It can be worn in your bra to fill it out after breast surgery.

- **Having breast reconstruction**, which is surgery that can rebuild the shape of a woman's breast, including her nipple and areola, the dark area around the nipple.

Some women are okay with having one breast or no breasts and do nothing. Other women feel better using breast forms to fill out their bras and make it look like they have two breasts when they wear clothes. Still other women have breast reconstruction, either right away or later. The choice is yours.

I may not want surgery to make a new breast. Without surgery, how can I look like I have two full breasts?

One option is wearing a breast form.

A breast form or prosthesis is usually heavy enough to match the weight of your remaining breast. It keeps your bra in place, helps your clothes fit better, and balances the weight of your other breast so you don't have backaches. Breast forms give you a natural look. Some can even be worn while you're swimming or exercising. They may be made of silicone, latex, or foam.

If you have had a double mastectomy, you can choose breast forms that will maintain a similar breast size.

If you have had a lumpectomy (breast-conserving surgery) or are small-breasted, you may only want a breast enhancer. They come in different sizes and shapes and are usually weighted a little bit. You can put one in your bra to make the breast on which you had surgery match the size of your other breast.

What should I know about a breast form?

You need to know how to find and pay for a breast form.[31]

- **Find out about costs.** Breast forms can be expensive. Insurance coverage of breast prostheses can vary. Check with your insurance company to see what is covered and how to submit claims. When buying bras or breast forms, mark "surgical" on your bills and any checks you write. Medicare and Medicaid will pay for some of these expenses if you are eligible.[31]

- **Ask your doctor for a prescription** for your breast form and any special bras. This prescription can help you get payment from your insurance company.

- **Find out whether you need a special bra.** Not every woman needs a special bra with a pocket to hold a breast form in place. Sometimes pockets can be added to bras you already have. Many stores sell pocket materials or precut pockets. Some will even sew pockets into your bras for you.

- **Make an appointment with a trained fitter** at the store before you go.

- **Try on different types of breast forms** while you're wearing a comfortable support bra. The most expensive breast form may not be the best fit for you.

- **Be sure the breast form matches your remaining breast** as closely as possible from the top, bottom, and front.

The American Cancer Society's "*tlc*" catalog sells breast forms and other products for women with cancer. To request a catalog or for more information on breast forms, call **800-850-9445**.

What Is Breast Reconstruction Surgery?

It is surgery to rebuild your breast.

Here's a list of possible breast reconstruction choices. Talk with your doctor about which choice might work best for you.

- **Breast implants:** An implant is a sac filled with saline (salt water) or silicone gel that the doctor puts under the muscle where the breast tissue was removed. This fills out the shape of your breast. This is the most common type of breast reconstruction. Sometimes reconstruction is done in stages over a few months if the skin over the breast needs to be stretched out with a temporary tissue expander first. Reconstruction may also be delayed until after radiation treatment is done. Both saline and silicone implants are safe.

Tissue expander

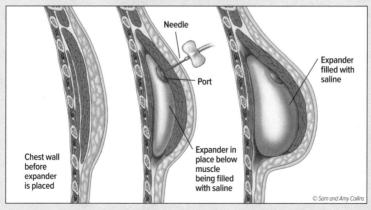

Needle

Port

Expander filled with saline

Chest wall before expander is placed

Expander in place below muscle being filled with saline

© Sam and Amy Collins

continued on next page

continued from previous page

- **Flap procedures:** A doctor uses tissue from somewhere else in your body to make what looks like a breast. The tissue can come from your lower belly (abdomen), back, hip, or buttocks.

Following are descriptions of different types of flap procedures.

The TRAM flap procedure uses tissue and muscle from the lower abdominal wall. The skin, fat, blood vessels, and muscle tissue are moved from the abdomen to the chest area. The flap is then shaped into the form of a breast. This results in less skin and fat in the lower belly (abdomen), or a "tummy tuck," although it can also cause some muscle weakness in the area.

The LAT flap procedure uses muscle and skin from your upper back. The muscle and skin are moved to your chest and shaped into a breast or, alternatively, into a "pocket" that can hold an implant. This type of flap is often used along with a breast implant.

The DIEP flap procedure uses fat and skin from the same area as the TRAM flap, but does not use the muscle to form the breast shape. It also results in a "tummy tuck."

The GAP flap procedure uses tissue from the buttocks to create the breast shape. It might be an option for women who can't or don't wish to use the abdominal sites, owing to thinness, incisions, failed abdominal flap, or other reasons, but it's not offered in many areas of the country.

Transverse rectus abdominis muscle (TRAM) flap

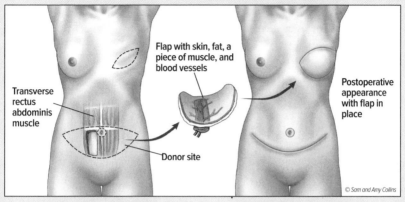

Flap with skin, fat, a piece of muscle, and blood vessels

Transverse rectus abdominis muscle

Donor site

Postoperative appearance with flap in place

© Sam and Amy Collins

This illustration depicts a free flap, in which the tissue is cut free from its original location and reattached in the chest area.

Latissimus dorsi muscle (LAT) flap

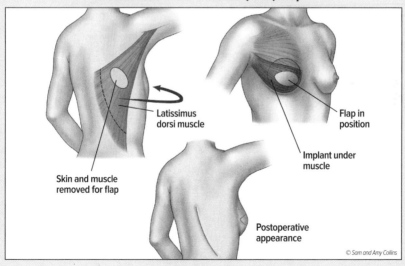

Latissimus dorsi muscle

Skin and muscle removed for flap

Flap in position

Implant under muscle

Postoperative appearance

© Sam and Amy Collins

continued on next page

continued from previous page

Deep inferior epigastric artery perforator (DIEP) flap

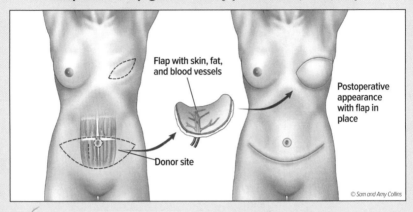

Flap with skin, fat, and blood vessels

Postoperative appearance with flap in place

Donor site

© Sam and Amy Collins

Gluteal free or Gluteal artery perforator (GAP) flap

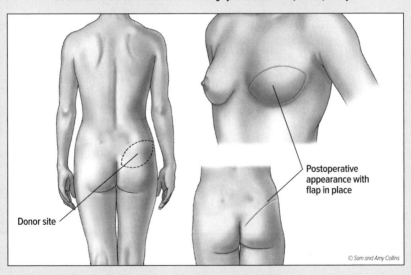

Donor site

Postoperative appearance with flap in place

© Sam and Amy Collins

Transverse upper gracilis (TUG) flap

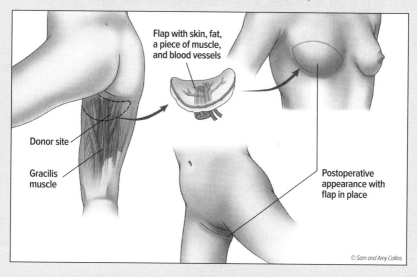

Flap with skin, fat, a piece of muscle, and blood vessels

Donor site

Gracilis muscle

Postoperative appearance with flap in place

© Sam and Amy Collins

The TUG flap procedure uses muscle and fatty tissue from along the bottom fold of the buttock extending to the inner thigh. It's only available in some centers.

• **Nipple reconstruction:** Tissue to create a new nipple and areola is often taken from your body, usually from the newly created breast or, less often, from another part of your body. Once the skin heals, a cosmetic procedure involving tattooing may be done to match the nipple of the other breast and to create the areola.

Can I have breast reconstruction surgery?

Most women can have surgery to rebuild the shape of their breasts.

You should be able to have this surgery whether you are young or older. If you think you want to have breast reconstruction, discuss it with your surgeon before you have your breast cancer surgery. Your doctor will probably want you to talk with a plastic surgeon as well. Talking about it early may give you more choices.

After you have spoken with your doctors about breast reconstruction, you may want to get a second opinion from another surgeon. You will want to choose which option will work best for you and your lifestyle.

What should I know about breast reconstruction?

Talk with your doctor about what to expect and the side effects you might have.

Ask your doctor questions about breast reconstruction. You also can talk to an American Cancer Society Reach To Recovery volunteer who has had breast reconstruction by calling **800-227-2345**. Keep in mind the following facts:

- **Breast reconstruction is expensive.** The Women's Health and Cancer Rights Act says that nearly all health plans that pay for mastectomies also have to pay for breast reconstruction. But you might still have to pay at least part of the costs, like a co-pay. Also, health plans must pay for prostheses.

  To find out more about your rights, call the U.S. Department of Labor (**866-444-3272**) or go online to **dol.gov/ebsa/publications/whcra.html**. Or call your State Insurance Commissioner's office. You can find the number online in the state government section.

- **Flap procedures leave scars** both where the tissue was taken and on the reconstructed breast.

- **Reconstruction won't make a "perfect" breast.** The goal of breast reconstruction is to make the size and shape of your breasts look alike so you'll feel comfortable when you wear clothes. You will be able to see the difference between your reconstructed breast and your other breast when you are naked.

- **Ask your doctor about his or her experience with different types of breast reconstruction.**

- **You will have less feeling in your reconstructed breast.** Nerves in the nipple and skin of your breast are affected by surgery.

? Questions

to ask the doctor about
breast reconstruction

1. Could I have breast reconstruction?

2. What types of reconstruction are available to me?

3. What is the average cost for each type?
   Does insurance cover these procedures?

4. What types of reconstruction might be best
   for me? Why?

5. What are the pros and cons of having
   reconstruction right away versus delaying it?

continued on next page

continued from previous page

6. Will I need more than one operation?

7. How should I expect the reconstructed breast to look?

8. Will I have any feeling in my reconstructed breast?

9. What possible side effects should I know about?

10. How much pain will I feel?

11. How long will I be in the hospital?

12. Will I need blood transfusions for the procedure? If so, can I donate my own blood?

13. How long will it take me to recover?

14. When would I be able to do things like driving and working?

15. What kinds of changes to my breast can I expect over time?

16. What happens to my breast as I get older, or if I gain or lose weight?

17. Are there any new reconstruction options that I should know about?

Is my cancer gone forever?

What if my cancer comes back?

Sometimes breast cancer does come back. You need to know that this doesn't happen to many women.

In some women, a few cancer cells live through treatment and grow into tumors. The cancer can recur (come back) where it first started or in your other breast. It also can come back in the lymph nodes close to the breast, or in other organs like the lungs, liver, brain, or bones. Here are some things to remember:

- **It's normal to worry about the chance that your cancer may come back.**

- **Don't wait to talk with your doctor** about anything happening in your body that worries you.

- **Everyone has aches and pains.** Most of the time, they aren't a sign that cancer is back. Call your doctor if the pain keeps getting worse or lasts for a few weeks.

- **Get regular checkups after treatment.** You'll probably feel better with each visit to your doctor. Your doctor can help you get on with your life without worrying too much about whether the cancer will come back.

Can I lower my chances that the cancer will come back?

Some medicines may lower your chance of breast cancer coming back.[11]

Depending on the stage of your cancer and other factors, your doctor might recommend chemotherapy or other treatments after surgery to help lower the risk of your cancer coming back. Exercise and nutrition (discussed on pages 147–150) are also important to help you stay healthy after treatment.

If your cancer was hormone-receptor positive (ER positive or PR positive), taking hormone therapy after your main treatment can help lower the chance that the cancer will come back. Because these drugs have side effects, you and your doctor will need to discuss them. Here are some medicines to discuss with your doctor:

- **Anastrozole (Arimidex), exemestane (Aromasin), and letrozole (Femara)** are newer, hormone-type medicines used to lower the risk of cancer coming back in women who have gone through menopause. These drugs can also cause side effects.

- **Tamoxifen (sold under the brand names Nolvadex, Istubal, and Valodex)** is also used to lower the risk that breast cancer will come back. Many studies show that taking tamoxifen for at least 5 years lowers a woman's chance of cancer coming back. Your doctor can tell you about side effects.[32]

How will I know if my cancer has come back?

See your doctor for regular checkups and tell him or her if you have new symptoms. This is the best way to find cancer that has come back.

If cancer does come back, it usually happens within a few years of a woman first finding out she has breast cancer. That is why it's so important after treatment to see your doctor on a regular schedule.[33] Follow these steps:

- **After treatment, look for any changes in your body.** Tell your doctor about anything new or strange. And pay attention to your own breasts. Tell your doctor about any lumps, bumps, or other changes you find.

- **Have a mammogram every year.** Having a mammogram is really important for women after breast cancer treatment. Some women may need a mammogram more often, as follow-up. If you have had certain kinds of mastectomy, you may not need to have mammograms on that side of your body anymore (although you still need them on the other breast). Ask your doctor.

When should I call the doctor?

Call the doctor about any changes you find or pain or other symptoms you have. Also, call if you have any questions.

Talk with your doctor about the following issues:

- Changes in your body you think might be a sign that cancer has come back

- Any pain you have

- Any problems that bother you or stop you from living your normal life. These include fatigue, trouble sleeping, not wanting to have sex, or gaining or losing weight.

- Any medicines, vitamins, or herbs you are taking, and any other treatments you are using

- Any strong feelings you have, like being worried or depressed

- Any changes in the health of your family

Questions
to ask the doctor about checkups
and cancer coming back

1. How often should I see you for checkups?

2. How will you check me for cancer?

3. What changes in my body should I watch for?

4. Will insurance cover my checkups?

5. Am I at high risk for my cancer coming back?

6. Is there anything I can do to lower the chances of my cancer coming back?

7. Could medicine help lower my chances of cancer coming back?

How can I be close with someone after cancer and treatment?

How will cancer and treatment affect my sex life?

It may take time for you to want to have sex again.

Many women find that they don't want to have sex during the time in which they're undergoing treatment. They may be thinking too much about other things. Some treatments may make you less interested in sex. See how you feel. Just know that it's okay to have sex if you want to.

You and your partner may need time to get used to being together again. Take the time you both need to feel relaxed. There are different ways to be close, like holding each other. After treatment, your partner may be afraid to have sex after everything you've gone through. You may need to be the one to say when you want to hug, kiss, and make love.

Talk about what you are afraid of or what bothers you. If you admit that you feel worried about being close or having sex, your partner may be able to give you the support you need. It may help if you both try these suggestions:

- Relax.
- Have fun.
- Be honest about how you feel.
- Talk about what the other person could do to make you feel better.
- Keep a sense of humor.

Should I talk about my cancer with someone new I'm dating?

Wait until you're comfortable with the person. Then be honest.

You may not want to talk about your cancer. Or you may worry that someone you're dating will not want to be with you because you've had cancer. Keep in mind the following:

- Telling a date within a few minutes of meeting is probably too soon. But if you wait until you are about to get into bed to tell a partner that you've had surgery on your breast, you risk shocking the person.

- Wait until you are both relaxed and feeling close to talk about your cancer.

- Share that you have had cancer if you get serious with someone, especially if cancer has affected how long you may live or whether you can have children.

Even people without cancer may reject each other because of looks, beliefs, personalities, or other reasons. Sadly, some dates may reject you because of your cancer. You could avoid being rejected if you stayed at home and didn't date. But you'd also miss the chance to be happy with someone. A loving partner will love you, regardless of your history.

How can I stay healthy from now on?

What can I do to keep my body healthy?

You can eat right and exercise, drink less, and not smoke.

You didn't have control over getting cancer, but you can do things to make your health better after cancer:

- Eat right.
- Exercise.
- Get to and stay at a healthy weight.
- Drink less alcohol, if you drink at all.
- Don't smoke.

Taking these steps is a good idea for anyone who wants to live a healthy life. We can't say for sure that taking these steps will keep your cancer from coming back, but they may help. And they can help keep you from getting another type of cancer.

How can I eat right after cancer treatment?

Eat a lot of healthy foods, like whole grains, vegetables, and fruits.

Being at a healthy weight is more important than ever. Eating a diet made up of mostly whole grains, vegetables, and fruits is good for your health and can help lower your cancer risk. And eating healthy will help you get to a healthy weight if you are overweight.

- Choose foods and drinks in amounts that help you maintain a healthy weight.
- Eat at least 2½ cups of vegetables and fruits each day.
- Choose whole grains instead of processed (refined) grains and sugars.
- Limit the amount of processed and red meats that you eat.

Low-fat and fat-free don't always mean low-calorie. Low-fat foods that are high in calories from sugar and other substances won't help you control your weight. Try eating whole grains, vegetables, and fruits instead of higher-calorie foods.

Eating right and being active go hand in hand. The key to weight control is to watch what you eat and how much you eat. Try to balance the calories you eat and drink with the calories you burn through exercise.

How should I exercise after cancer treatment?

Talk with your doctor first. Find out what kinds of exercise are safe for you. Then have fun.

Exercise can help you feel like you're in charge of your body again. It also can help you feel good about reaching your activity goals. Exercise can help you build stronger muscles, become more flexible, and have more energy. You may feel more relaxed and positive after exercising. Follow these tips[34,35]:

- **Avoid inactivity and return to normal daily activities as soon as possible following diagnosis.**

- **Don't overdo it.** If you haven't exercised in a while, start slowly with just a few minutes a day. You will get stronger. Talk with your doctor to find out what kinds of exercise are safe and healthy for you.

- **Try to be active for at least 150 minutes each week.** Have fun and pick exercises you like. This will help you stick with a plan and reach your activity goals.

- **Include strength training at least 2 days per week.**

- **Do your exercise; slow down before you stop to cool down.** And, while your muscles are still warm, stretch before you stop.

- **Try different exercises** like walking, swimming, lifting weights, and yoga. It's good to mix exercises that build strength (lifting weights) with those that get your heart pumping faster (walking or swimming).

- **Talk with a doctor or physical therapist about your risk of lymphedema before you start exercising.** Find out whether different types of exercise might make your risk higher and how to protect against lymphedema. (See pages 76–78 to read more about lymphedema.)

Call the American Cancer Society at **800-227-2345** for more information on eating healthy and staying active.[34,35]

How can I get back to living my life?

Can I live a normal life again?

You can live a full and happy life after treatment.

You are a woman who has had cancer, but there is more to your life than that. Doing the things that have always made you happy may make you feel better and more normal now. If you feel like it, go out and enjoy yourself.

After dealing with breast cancer and treatment, you may feel tired. You may have forgotten what it was like to just do things you enjoy. Try some of the ideas below to feel normal again and make yourself happy.

Express yourself:

- **Laugh.** Watch a funny movie or spend time with a friend who makes you smile.

- **Share your thoughts and feelings** by painting, writing in a journal, singing, or dancing.

- **Talk with someone you trust.** Find someone you feel safe with—a partner, friend, sister, religious leader, or counselor—and really let out your thoughts and feelings.

Do things for you:

- **Work your mind.** Read a book, take a class, or try a new hobby.

- **Take time alone.** Set a time each day or week to do just what you want to do.

- **Do nice things for yourself.** Check out books from the library, rent a movie, ask your partner to give you a foot massage, or take a hot bath.

Think about what's important:

- **Decide what really matters** and let go of the "small stuff."

- **Tap into your faith.** Join a prayer group at your place of worship if you belong to one. Find prayers you like and say them often.

- **Set limits.** Think about your work, your chores around the house, and your social life. Then set some limits. Cut back on activities until you are doing only what matters most and what brings you the most rewards.

What do I do now?

You decide what happens in your life now.

Sometimes having cancer makes people think about their lives in a different way. You may not worry so much about small problems. You may want to spend more time with the people you love and less time at work or doing housework. Or you may realize how important your family, job, free time, or friendships are to you.

Think about coming up with a list of simple things you can do to make your life better. Be specific. Here are some ideas:

- Call a loved one once a week.
- Volunteer with a cancer support group one day a month.
- Learn to dance, paint, or play an instrument.
- Read a book you've always wanted to read.
- Plan a vacation to a beautiful place.
- Go visit an old friend.
- Spend an hour by yourself once a week and do whatever you want.
- Eat a family dinner together 3 nights a week with no TV.

Cancer may have shown you that each day you are alive is a gift. It is up to you to make each day what you want it to be.

More Information

Can you help me understand breast cancer risk?

What does it mean if I am "at risk" for breast cancer?

Being "at risk" for breast cancer has to do with things that raise your chances of getting breast cancer.[2]

A risk factor is something in your life that raises your chance of something happening, like getting breast cancer. Any woman could get breast cancer, but the things listed on page 156 can raise a woman's chances of getting it.

The idea of risk factors can be confusing. Just because a woman has one or more risk factors for breast cancer doesn't mean that she will get breast cancer. Even if risk factors raise the chances that breast cancer could grow, they don't mean that it *will* grow.

What risk factors raise a woman's chances of getting breast cancer?

There are 2 kinds of risk factors that can raise a woman's chances of getting breast cancer.

The first type of risk factor is something that a woman can't change. Here are some examples:

- Being a woman
- Getting older
- Having a close relative (sister, mother, child, father, or brother) who has had breast cancer
- Having an inherited mutation in a *BRCA* gene (or certain other genes)
- Going through menopause at a later age

The second type of risk factor is related to lifestyle. Here are some examples:

- Not having children
- Having a first child after the age of 30
- Using birth control pills
- Drinking 2 or more drinks of alcohol a day
- Taking combined hormone therapy after menopause
- Being overweight or obese

Are other women in my family more likely to get breast cancer?

Your mother, sisters, or daughters do have a higher chance of getting breast cancer.

A small portion of breast cancers "run in families." This means that if one woman in your family has breast cancer, the other women in your family have a greater chance of getting it, too. If, in addition to you, your mother, sister, or daughter also has breast cancer, the risk is even higher for your other female relatives. The risk is also higher if anyone was diagnosed with breast cancer before age 50.

If this describes your family, tell your close female relatives to talk with their doctors. Doctors may want them to start having mammograms and other tests when they are young. See also pages 38–39 for information on genetic counseling.

Remember, the fact that you have breast cancer doesn't mean that other members of your family will get it. It means that their risk is higher than that of women without breast cancer in their families.

Can anything lower a person's chances of getting breast cancer?

Yes. Some things may lower the risk of getting breast cancer.

If you have breast cancer, you may want to know how to help your friends and loved ones lower their risk of getting breast cancer. These tips also may help lower your risk of having breast cancer come back after treatment.

Here are some guidelines:

- Keep a healthy weight instead of being overweight.
- Exercise each day.
- Drink less alcohol.
- Eat lots of fruits and vegetables and less red meat.

Living a healthy life can help a woman lower her chances of getting breast cancer. It doesn't mean she won't get breast cancer, but it might help. And taking the steps above also helps lower her chances of getting certain other cancers, as well as heart disease, diabetes, and some other health problems.

I've heard that breast implants can raise your chances of getting breast cancer. Is that true?

Many of the beliefs people have about what causes breast cancer are not true[36]:

- **Breast implants:** Breast implants don't raise breast cancer risk.

- **Abortion or miscarriage:** Having an abortion or a miscarriage has not been shown to raise the risk of breast cancer.

- **Antiperspirants:** Using underarm antiperspirants or regular deodorants has not been shown to raise risk.

- **Getting hurt:** A breast injury does not raise cancer risk.

- **Underwire bras:** Bras with underwires don't raise breast cancer risk.

How can I have breast cancer if no one in my family has had it?

Women who don't have a family member with breast cancer can still get breast cancer.

Women who don't have a close relative with breast cancer may still get breast cancer. In fact, most breast cancer occurs in women who don't have any other close family member with it. You may be the first person in your family to get breast cancer.

More about cancer stages

On my pathology report, what do the letters T, N, and M and the numbers 0, 1, 2, 3, and 4 mean?

These letters and numbers are part of a staging system that describes how much and where the cancer has spread in your body.

The letters T, N, and M are used to describe the size of your tumor and how much the cancer has grown or spread.

- **T** stands for the size of the breast tumor and whether it has grown into nearby structures.
- **N** stands for any cancer that has spread to the lymph nodes near the breast. (Lymph nodes are small, bean-shaped areas of tissue that help fight infections in the body.)
- **M** stands for cancer that has spread to other parts of the body (like the bones, lungs, brain, or liver).

Numbers follow each of these letters. Lower numbers mean you have a smaller tumor or a tumor that has not spread much or at all. Higher numbers mean you have a larger tumor or a tumor that has spread more.

- **T0, Tis, T1, T2, T3, and T4:** T0 represents no evidence of a primary tumor. Tis (cancer in situ) means the cancer cells have not grown deeply into the breast tissue. T1, T2, and T3 account for invasive breast tumors of increasing size, while T4 represents cancer of any size that has spread to the chest wall or the skin.

- **N0, N1, N2, and N3:** N0 represents no spread to the nearby lymph nodes and is the least serious. N3 has spread widely to the lymph nodes and is the most serious.

- **M0 and M1:** M0 means the cancer has not spread to other areas of the body, and M1 means cancer has spread to other areas.

- **TX, NX, and MX** are used if a tumor, lymph nodes, or distant spread can't be assessed.

My doctor says I have stage IIIA breast cancer. How are the letters T, N, and M and the numbers 0 to 4 related to the stage?

They are related. Doctors use the T, N, and M categories to figure out one number and letter that describes your cancer stage, like IIIA.

Doctors will look at each of the T, N, and M categories of your cancer before deciding on the overall stage of your cancer.

When doctors figure out your overall cancer stage, they don't talk about the T, N, and M categories. They use a shortcut: a single Roman numeral (and often a letter).

Every woman's breast cancer is said to be one of these stages: stage 0 (Tis, in situ), stage IA, stage IB, stage IIA, stage IIB, stage IIIA, stage IIIB, stage IIIC, or stage IV.

Ask your doctor what your cancer stage means for your health, your treatment options, and your future.

What's the difference between my stage IIB breast cancer and my friend's stage IIIB breast cancer?

Breast cancer is more advanced if it is described by a higher stage number and letter.

Someone whose cancer has grown and spread a lot will have higher numbers in the T, N, and possibly M categories. Her cancer also will be a higher overall stage. This means she has a more advanced cancer than someone whose cancer has not grown and spread as much (and who has a lower overall stage). Here are some examples:

- Someone whose cancer is T2, N1, and M0 has stage IIB breast cancer.

- Someone whose cancer is T4, N2, M0 has stage IIIB breast cancer. She has a more advanced cancer than a woman with stage IIB breast cancer. Her T number, which means her tumor size, and N number, which has to do with whether the cancer has spread to lymph nodes, are more advanced than the T and N numbers of the woman with stage IIB breast cancer.

Your Medical Team

You will have many health professionals and support staff working with you during your breast cancer diagnosis, treatment, and recovery. Here's a list of some of the people who might be members of your cancer care team (although you might not need all of them):

Anesthesiologist

This is a medical doctor who gives anesthesia drugs to put you to sleep for surgery or other procedures. These drugs also help prevent or relieve pain during and after surgery.

Genetic Counselor

This type of counselor is trained to help people through the process of genetic testing. A genetic counselor can explain the available tests, discuss the pros and cons of testing, and address any concerns you may have. This counselor can also arrange for genetic testing and help interpret results.

Medical Oncologist

An expert in cancer care and treatment, this doctor will help you make decisions about your treatment and will be in charge of your cancer treatment (like chemotherapy or hormone therapy) if they are needed. He or she may stay in touch with other members of your medical team to make sure you get the best treatment possible. Your oncologist will follow up with you during your treatments.

Nurses

Several different nurses may care for patients with breast cancer. A registered nurse can monitor your condition, give treatment, tell you about side effects, and help you adjust to the effects of breast cancer. A nurse practitioner (NP) shares many tasks with your doctors, such as recording your medical history, giving physical exams, doing follow-up care, and writing prescriptions (with the doctor's supervision). A clinical nurse specialist (CNS) may provide special services, such as leading support groups. An oncology nurse has a great deal of knowledge about cancer care and may work in several areas.

Occupational Therapist (OT)

This health care professional works with people with impairments or limitations to help them develop and recover skills needed for daily living.

Pain Specialist

These are doctors, nurses, and pharmacists who are experts in managing pain. They can help you find pain control that works and helps you maintain your quality of life. Not all doctors and nurses are trained in pain care, so you may have to request a pain specialist if your pain relief needs are not being met.

Pathologist

This is a doctor who has been trained to diagnose disease by looking at tissue and fluid samples. He or she will determine the cell type and grade of your cancer and write a pathology report so that you and your doctor can decide on treatment options.

Primary Care Physician

This may be a general doctor or one with special training in gynecology, internal medicine, or family practice. He or she is often the doctor who screened you for breast cancer. This doctor will talk with you about your breast cancer and will be involved in your care. Your primary care physician provides details of your medical history to other members of the team. He or she also will refer you to breast cancer care specialists.

Physical Therapist (PT)

A physical therapist helps you regain strength and movement after surgery. The physical therapist teaches you exercises and other ways to strengthen your body. He or she may use massage or heat to help you restore or maintain your body's strength, function, and flexibility.

Plastic/Reconstructive Surgeon

This is a medical doctor who operates to restore parts of the body affected by injury, disease, or treatments for cancer. You may talk with him or her before and after breast cancer surgery. Your plastic or reconstructive surgeon can perform breast reconstruction during or after a mastectomy.

Psychiatrist or Psychologist

As a medical doctor specializing in mental health and behavioral disorders, a psychiatrist provides counseling and can also prescribe medicine.

A psychologist is a licensed mental health professional who may be part of your medical team. He or she provides counseling on emotional and psychological issues. A psychologist may have special training and experience in treating people with cancer.

Radiation Oncologist

A radiation oncologist is a medical doctor who treats cancer with radiation (high-energy x-rays). He or she will decide what kind and how much radiation you should get after your breast-conserving surgery or mastectomy, or to control advanced breast cancer. This member of your medical team checks on you often during and after treatment.

Radiation Therapist

A radiation therapist is a trained technician who works with the radiation oncologist (see previous page). He or she positions your body during the treatment and gives you the radiation therapy.

Radiologist

This is a medical doctor who has special training in using x-rays, mammography, ultrasound, and other imaging procedures. He or she has special training in diagnosing breast cancer and other diseases. Your radiologist writes a radiology report to your personal doctor, medical oncologist, radiation oncologist, or surgeon describing the findings. The radiology images and report may be used to aid in diagnosis, help locate tumors during surgery and radiation treatment, or help classify the stage (extent) of your breast cancer.

Radiologic Technologist

This person assists the radiologist. He or she is trained to position you for x-rays and mammograms and to develop and check the images for quality. The images taken by your radiology technologist are sent to your radiologist to be read.

Registered Dietitian

A registered dietitian (RD) helps you make healthy diet choices and maintain a healthy weight before, during, and after cancer treatment.

Social Worker

A social worker can help you and your family deal with emotional and practical problems, like finances, child care, emotional issues, family concerns and relationships, transportation, and problems with the health care system. Your social worker may have special training in cancer-related problems and can provide counseling, answer questions about treatment, and lead cancer support groups.

Surgeon or Surgical Oncologist

This is a medical doctor who performs surgery. You will consult with your surgeon before and after you have a biopsy, breast-conserving surgery, mastectomy, or other surgical procedure. The surgeon will remove tumors and, if necessary, surrounding tissue. Your surgeon works closely with other members of your medical team. He or she will give a surgical report to your doctor and to your radiation and medical oncologists that will help plan your future treatment.

References

1. American Cancer Society. *Cancer Treatment and Survivorship Facts & Figures 2016-2017.* Atlanta: American Cancer Society; 2016.

2. American Cancer Society. Detailed guide: Breast cancer. What are the risk factors for breast cancer? cancer.org/cancer/breastcancer/detailedguide/breast-cancer-risk-factors. Last modified February 26, 2015, accessed May 21, 2015.

3. American Cancer Society. The possibility of facing cancer again/Advanced and metastatic cancer. In: O'Regan R, Gabram-Mendola SGA, Ades T, Alteri R, Kramer J, Stump-Sutliff KA, eds. *Breast Cancer Journey: The Essential Guide to Treatment and Recovery.* Third Edition. Atlanta: American Cancer Society; 2013:75,422.

4. American Cancer Society. Making the medical system work for you/Getting a second opinion. In: O'Regan R, Gabram-Mendola SGA, Ades T, Alteri R, Kramer J, Stump-Sutliff KA, eds. *Breast Cancer Journey: The Essential Guide to Treatment and Recovery.* Third Edition. Atlanta: American Cancer Society; 2013:109–111.

5. American Cancer Society. Making the medical system work for you/Your medical team. In: O'Regan R, Gabram-Mendola SGA, Ades T, Alteri R, Kramer J, Stump-Sutliff KA, eds. *Breast Cancer Journey: The Essential Guide to Treatment and Recovery.* Third Edition. Atlanta: American Cancer Society; 2013:101–106.

6. American Cancer Society. Who gets breast cancer? In: O'Regan R, Gabram-Mendola SGA, Ades T, Alteri R, Kramer J, Stump-Sutliff KA, eds. *Breast Cancer Journey: The Essential Guide to Treatment and Recovery.* Third Edition. Atlanta: American Cancer Society; 2013:22,23.

7. James ML, Lehman M, Hider PN, Jeffery M, Hickey BE, Francis DP. Fraction size in radiation treatment for breast conservation in early breast cancer. *Cochrane Database Syst Rev.* 2010 Nov 10;(11):CD003860. doi:10.1002/14651858. CD003860. pub3.

8. Haviland JS, Owen JR, Dewar JA, et al; START Trialists' Group. The UK Standardisation of Breast Radiotherapy (START) trials of radiotherapy hypofractionation for treatment of early breast cancer: 10-year follow-up results of two randomised controlled trials. *Lancet Oncol.* 2013 Oct;14(11):1086–1094. Epub 2013 Sep 19.

9. Smith BD, Bentzen SM, Correa CR, et al. Fractionation for whole breast irradiation: an American Society for Radiation Oncology (ASTRO) evidence-based guideline. *Int J Radiat Oncol Biol Phys.* 2011;81(1):59.

10. American Cancer Society. Other treatments for breast cancer/Chemotherapy. In: O'Regan R, Gabram-Mendola SGA, Ades T, Alteri R, Kramer J, Stump-Sutliff KA, eds. *Breast Cancer Journey: The Essential Guide to Treatment and Recovery.* Third Edition. Atlanta: American Cancer Society; 2013:168–177.

11. American Cancer Society. Other treatments for breast cancer/Hormone therapy. In: O'Regan R, Gabram-Mendola SGA, Ades T, Alteri R, Kramer J, Stump-Sutliff KA, eds. *Breast Cancer Journey: The Essential Guide to Treatment and Recovery.* Third Edition. Atlanta: American Cancer Society; 2013:183–188.

12. American Cancer Society. Other treatments for breast cancer/Targeted therapy. In: O'Regan R, Gabram-Mendola SGA, Ades T, Alteri R, Kramer J, Stump-Sutliff KA, eds. *Breast Cancer Journey: The Essential Guide to Treatment and Recovery.* Third Edition. Atlanta: American Cancer Society; 2013:188–192.

13. American Cancer Society. Other treatments for breast cancer/Drugs to protect the bones. In: O'Regan R, Gabram-Mendola SGA, Ades T, Alteri R, Kramer J, Stump-Sutliff KA, eds. *Breast Cancer Journey: The Essential Guide to Treatment and Recovery.* Third Edition. Atlanta: American Cancer Society; 2013:192–193.

14. American Cancer Society. *American Cancer Society Complete Guide to Complementary & Alternative Cancer Therapies.* Second Edition. Atlanta: American Cancer Society; 2009.

15. American Cancer Society. Coping with symptoms and side effects. In: O'Regan R, Gabram-Mendola SGA, Ades T, Alteri R, Kramer J, Stump-Sutliff KA, eds. *Breast Cancer Journey: The Essential Guide to Treatment and Recovery.* Third Edition. Atlanta: American Cancer Society; 2013:247–285.

16. Shah C, Vicini FA. Breast cancer-related arm lymphedema: incidence rates, diagnostic techniques, optimal management and risk reduction strategies. *J Radiat Oncol Biol Phys.* 2011;81:907–914. doi: 10.1016/j.ijrobp.2011.05.043. Epub 2011 Sep 22.

17. Norman SA, Localio AR, Potashnik SL, et al. Lymphedema in breast cancer survivors: incidence, degree, time course, treatment, and symptoms. *J Clin Oncol.* 2009;27:390–397.

18. American Cancer Society. Coping with symptoms and side effects/ Lymphedema. In: O'Regan R, Gabram-Mendola SGA, Ades T, Alteri R, Kramer J, Stump-Sutliff KA, eds. *Breast Cancer Journey: The Essential Guide to Treatment and Recovery.* Third Edition. Atlanta: American Cancer Society; 2013:276–285.

19. American Cancer Society. Acupuncture. cancer.org/treatment/ treatmentsandsideeffects/physicalsideeffects/pain/paindiary/pain-control-acupuncture. Last revised July 15, 2015, accessed July 16, 2015.

20. National Cancer Institute. About Cancer/Acupuncture. cancer.gov/about-cancer/treatment/cam/patient/acupuncture-pdq/#link/_57. Accessed July 16, 2015.

21. Cramer H, Lauche R, Paul A, Langhorst J, Kümmel S, Dobos GJ. Hypnosis in breast cancer care: a systematic review of randomized controlled trials. *Integr Cancer Ther.* 2015 Jan;14(1):5–15. doi: 10.1177/1534735415550035. Epub 2014 Sep 18.

22. Marchand L. Integrative and complementary therapies for patients with advanced cancer. *Ann Palliat Med.* 2014;3(3):160–171. doi: 10.3978/J. issn.2224-5820.2014.07.01.

23. Simon S. Open enrollment under way for health care law. cancer.org/cancer/news/news/open-enrollment-begins-for-health-care-law. November 6, 2014.

24. American Cancer Society, National Endowment for Financial Education. Treatment: Financial Guidance for Cancer Survivors and Their Families. No.350001. cancer.org/acs/groups/content/@editorial/documents/document/acsq-020182.pdf. Last modified February 2014, accessed May 22, 2015.

25. American Cancer Society. Coping with your diagnosis and moving forward. In: O'Regan R, Gabram-Mendola SGA, Ades T, Alteri R, Kramer J, Stump-Sutliff KA, eds. *Breast Cancer Journey: The Essential Guide to Treatment and Recovery.* Third Edition. Atlanta: American Cancer Society; 2013:85–92.

26. Simard S, Savard J, Ivers H. Fear of cancer recurrence: specific profiles and nature of intrusive thoughts. *J Cancer Surviv.* 2010;4(4):361–371. doi: 10.1007/s11764-010-0136-8. Epub 2010 Jul 10.

27. Tomich PL, Helgeson VS. Five years later: a cross-sectional comparison of breast cancer survivors with healthy women. *Psychooncology.* 2002;11(2):154–169.

28. Heiney SP, Hermann JF. *Cancer in Our Family: Helping Children Cope with a Parent's Illness.* Second Edition. Atlanta: American Cancer Society; 2013.

29. Fullbright CD. *How to Help Your Friend with Cancer.* Atlanta: American Cancer Society; 2015.

30. American Cancer Society. Employment and workplace issues. In: O'Regan R, Gabram-Mendola SGA, Ades T, Alteri R, Kramer J, Stump-Sutliff KA, eds. *Breast Cancer Journey: The Essential Guide to Treatment and Recovery.* Third Edition. Atlanta: American Cancer Society; 2013:323–327.

31. American Cancer Society. Breast reconstruction and prostheses. In: O'Regan R, Gabram-Mendola SGA, Ades T, Alteri R, Kramer J, Stump-Sutliff KA, eds. *Breast Cancer Journey: The Essential Guide to Treatment and Recovery.* Third Edition. Atlanta: American Cancer Society; 2013:319.

32. American Cancer Society. Hormone therapy for breast cancer. cancer.org/cancer/breastcancer/detailedguide/breast-cancer-treating-hormone-therapy. Last modified June 10, 2015, accessed August 11, 2015.

33. Runowicz CD, Leach CR, Henry NL, et al. American Cancer Society/American Society of Clinical Oncology Breast Cancer Survivorship Care Guideline. *CA Cancer J Clin.* 2016;66(1):43–73. doi: 10 3322/caac. 21319. Epub 2015 Dec 7.

34. Rock CL, Doyle C, Demark-Wahnefried W, et al. Nutrition and physical activity guidelines for cancer survivors. *CA Cancer J Clin.* 2012;62(4):243–274. doi: 10 3322/caac. 21142. Epub 2012 Apr 26. Erratum in *CA Cancer J Clin.* 2013;63(3):215.

35. Grant BL, Bloch AS, Hamilton KK, Thomson CA. *American Cancer Society Complete Guide to Nutrition for Cancer Survivors.* Second Edition. Atlanta: American Cancer Society; 2010.

36. American Cancer Society. Who gets breast cancer? In: O'Regan R, Gabram-Mendola SGA, Ades T, Alteri R, Kramer J, Stump-Sutliff KA, eds. *Breast Cancer Journey: The Essential Guide to Treatment and Recovery.* Third Edition. Atlanta: American Cancer Society; 2013:32,33.

Resource Guide

Listed on pages 176–183 are resources from the American Cancer Society, as well as other organizations that you may find helpful. You may also find specific breast cancer support services in your area. Ask your doctor or check with your local hospital or the Internet for nearby sources of help.

There is endless information about cancer and related topics on the Internet. This can be helpful when you are choosing what to do about your health. But think about where the information comes from. Is the group giving the information respected? Can you trust what they say? Are they trying to sell you something? Always talk with your doctor about health information you find on the Internet. He or she can help you figure out if you can trust the information.

American Cancer Society Programs and Services

American Cancer Society
Toll-free number: 800-227-2345
Website: cancer.org

The **American Cancer Society (ACS)** provides educational materials, information, and patient services to help people with cancer and their loved ones understand cancer, manage their lives through treatment and recovery, and find the emotional support they need. A comprehensive resource for all your cancer-related questions, the Society can also put you in touch with community resources in your area.

American Cancer Society National Cancer Information Center (NCIC)

The NCIC provides information and support to those facing cancer 24 hours a day, 365 days a year. Trained cancer information specialists are available to provide accurate, up-to-date cancer information to patients, family members, and caregivers and connect them with valuable services and resources in their communities.

Toll-free Line: 800-227-2345

American Cancer Society Patient Navigator Program

The American Cancer Society Patient Navigator Program matches individuals with a trained patient navigator at a cancer treatment center. Navigators work one-on-one with patients to connect them to helpful programs and services, as well as listening and providing support in times of need. Call the toll-free number, 800-227-2345, to learn more about this program.

Health Insurance Assistance Service (HIAS)

HIAS provides guidance to cancer patients, cancer survivors, and caregivers about health insurance options that are available through the Affordable Care Act open enrollment. To learn more, call the toll-free number, 800-227-2345, and ask for an HIAS representative.

Patient Lodging Programs

Getting the best care sometimes means cancer patients must travel away from home. This can place an extra emotional and financial burden on patients and caregivers during an already challenging time. The American Cancer Society is trying to make this difficult situation easier for both cancer patients and their families through **Hope Lodge®** and our **Hotel Partners Program**.

There are more than 30 Hope Lodge locations throughout the United States, and more lodges are being built. Accommodations and eligibility requirements may vary by location. To find out more about a Hope Lodge, please go to cancer.org, select **Find Local Resources**, and choose a location from the list there, or enter your zip code on the page. If there is not a Hope Lodge in your area, please call the toll-free number, 800-227-2345, for more information.

Road To Recovery® (Rides to treatment)

Every day, cancer patients need rides to treatment. Some may not be able to drive themselves, and family and friends can't always help. The ACS Road To Recovery program provides rides to patients who have no way to get to their cancer treatment centers.

Volunteer drivers donate their time and the use of their cars so that patients can receive the lifesaving treatments they need. If you or your loved one needs a ride to treatment, call the American Cancer Society at 800-227-2345 to be matched with a volunteer, or go to cancer.org, search for Road To Recovery, and enter your zip code in the space provided.

Relay For Life®

Relay For Life®, the American Cancer Society's signature event, is designed to bring together those who have been touched by cancer. Relay participants help raise money and awareness to support the American Cancer Society in its lifesaving mission to eliminate cancer as a major health issue.

Website: relayforlife.org/relay

American Cancer Society Cancer Action Network℠ (ACS CAN)

ACS CAN is all about ensuring that fighting cancer is a top priority for our lawmakers. All ACS CAN members are notified of cancer-related issues pending in government agencies.

Website: acscan.org

Online Support Programs

American Cancer Society Cancer Survivors Network® (ACSCSN)

ACSCSN is a community of cancer survivors, families, and friends who have been touched by cancer. The website provides a private, secure way to find and communicate with others to share personal views, feelings, and experiences. Content is not endorsed by the American Cancer Society nor should it be accepted as credible medical information. Users are encouraged to visit the American Cancer Society website at cancer.org, or call 800-227-2345 for credible medical information. Users should always consult qualified health care providers with questions and concerns about their medical condition.

Website: cancer.org/csn

MyLifeLine.org

With MyLifeLine.org, cancer patients and caregivers can connect with family and friends, allowing them to share their cancer journey, get support, and focus on healing. When you set up a free webpage, you can share updates and photos with selected family and friends in one secure place; get the help you need by organizing meals, rides to treatment, and more through the Helping Calendar; feel empowered by messages of love and support from friends and family; and review and share cancer resources vetted by experts. These free personalized webpages will help empower your family and friends to be a stronger support community for you.

Website: acs.mylifelineorg

Other Support Programs

Look Good Feel Better (Help with appearance–related side effects of treatment)

In a Look Good Feel Better session, trained volunteer cosmetologists teach women, men, and teens how to cope with skin changes and hair loss by using cosmetics and skin care products donated by the cosmetic industry. To find a program near you, go to the Look Good Feel Better website and enter your zip code in the space provided. To speak with someone by phone, call the toll-free number (below), or contact the American Cancer Society at 800-227-2345 for more information.

Website: lookgoodfeelbetter.org

Toll-free Line: 800-395-LOOK (800-395-5665)

Reach To Recovery® (Breast cancer support)

Women with breast cancer may want to talk to someone who knows what they are feeling—someone who has "been there." Through the Reach To Recovery program, breast cancer patients are matched with a volunteer who will talk with them about coping with breast cancer diagnosis and treatment.

Reach To Recovery volunteers are specially trained to help people through their experience by offering a measure of comfort and an opportunity for emotional grounding and informed decision making. As breast cancer survivors, our volunteers give patients and family members an opportunity to express feelings, talk about fears and concerns, and ask questions. Program volunteers do not provide medical advice.

To be matched with a volunteer, call the toll-free number, 800-227-2345, or go to cancer.org, search for **Reach To Recovery**, and enter your zip code in the space provided.

"*tlc*" (Hair loss and mastectomy products)

"*tlc*" is the American Cancer Society's catalog and website for women coping with the appearance-related effects of cancer. It offers helpful information and affordable products, including wigs, hairpieces, breast forms, mastectomy bras, hats, turbans, mastectomy swimwear, and accessories. All proceeds from product sales are reinvested into the American Cancer Society's programs and services for patients and survivors.

Website: tlcdirect.org

To order products or catalogs: 800-850-9445

General Cancer Information and Support

Government agencies and organizations are also available to provide information and support. You may also find support services in your local area. Ask your doctor, check with your hospital, or search the Internet for nearby sources of help.

National Cancer Institute (NCI)

The National Cancer Institute (NCI) provides information on cancer research, diagnosis, and treatment to patients and health care providers. Callers are automatically connected to the office serving their region. The service offers free publications and the opportunity to speak directly with a cancer specialist who can provide information on treatment and make appropriate referrals. NCI also offers a comprehensive database, "National Organizations That Offer Cancer-Related Support Services."

Website: cancer.gov

Toll-free Line: 800-4-CANCER (800-422-6237)

TTY: 800-332-8615

Centers for Disease Control and Prevention (CDC)

CDC is a leader in nationwide efforts to ease the burden of cancer. Basic information and statistics about some of the most common cancers in the United States can be found on the CDC's website. Through the Division of Cancer Prevention and Control (DCPC), CDC works with national cancer organizations, state health agencies, and other key groups to develop, implement, and promote effective strategies for preventing and controlling cancer.

Website: cdc.gov/cancer

Toll-free Line: 800-CDC-INFO (800-232-4636)

Medicare Hotline

The Medicare hotline offers information about who can be part of Medicare, how to sign up, what is covered, payment and billing, insurance, prescription drugs, and frequently asked questions. Call to get information about services in your area.

U.S. Department of Health & Human Services

Website: medicare.gov

Toll-free Line: 800-MEDICAR (800-633-4227)

U.S. Social Security Administration

The Social Security Administration runs the Supplemental Security Income (SSI) program. They can tell you how to apply for Social Security Disability Income (SSDI). Breast cancer could qualify you for disability.

Website: ssa.gov

Toll-free Line: 800-772-1213

Hill-Burton Free and Reduced–Cost Health Care

U.S. Department of Health and Human Services

Health Resources and Services Administration

Depending on the size of your family and how much money you make, you may be able to get help paying for your health care through the Hill-Burton program. You can apply for Hill-Burton at any time, before or after you have care.

Hill-Burton facilities must post a sign in their admissions and business offices and emergency room that says: NOTICE—Medical Care for Those Who Cannot Afford to Pay. They must provide you a written list of the types of services that are eligible for Hill-Burton free or reduced-cost care, what income level qualifies for free or reduced-cost care, and how long the facility may take in determining an applicant's eligibility.

Only facility costs are covered—not your private doctors' bills. Some facilities may use different eligibility standards and procedures. For example, they may require you to provide documentation that verifies your eligibility, like proof of income.

To find a Hill-Burton facility near you, go to the website below and enter your zip code in the space provided, or call the toll-free number. Then ask to speak to someone in the admissions, business, or patient accounts office there. They can tell you how to apply for Hill-Burton.

Toll-free Line: 800-638-0742

Toll-free in Maryland: 800-492-0359

Website: hrsa.gov/gethealthcare/affordable/hillburton

Glossary

areola *(ah-REE-uh-luh or air-ee-O-luh)*: the dark area around the nipple.

benign *(be-NINE)*: not cancer. Tumors can be either cancer or benign. Not all lumps or tumors are cancer; some are benign.

axillary lymph node *(AX-ill-air-ee limf node)*: a lymph node in the armpit.

axillary lymph node dissection *(AX-ill-air-ee limf node di-SEK-shun)*: removal of the lymph nodes in the armpit (axillary nodes). They are examined under a microscope to determine whether they contain cancer. See also *lymph nodes.*

biopsy *(BY-op-see)*: taking out some tissue, such as from the lump in your breast. Doctors look at the sample of tissue and cells under a microscope to find out whether a person has cancer and to learn more about it.

bone-directed therapy: a type of therapy that uses medicines to help strengthen bones and may prevent the spread of cancer to the bone.

brachytherapy *(BRAY-kee-THAIR-uh-pee)*: internal radiation treatment given by placing radioactive material directly into the tumor or close to it.

breast cancer: cancer that starts in the breast. Cancer cells in the breast are growing and forming new cells without stopping or dying like healthy cells do.

breast-conserving surgery: treatment aimed at saving or conserving the breast; it involves having a lumpectomy (and usually radiation therapy).

breast form: also called a prosthesis. It is padding shaped like a breast or part of a breast that can be worn in your bra to fill it out after breast surgery.

breast implant: a flexible sac filled with saline (salt water) or silicone gel that is put just under the skin where breast tissue was removed. This fills out the shape of your breast.

breast reconstruction: surgery that rebuilds the shape of a woman's breast, including her nipple and areola.

cancer: a group of diseases that cause cells in the body to change and grow out of control. Healthy cells in your body grow, form new cells, do what they are supposed to do in your body, and later die. But cancer cells keep growing, forming more cells, and spreading in the body. They don't die like other cells.

cancer grade: how abnormal your cancer cells look compared with normal cells. Cancers with higher grades tend to grow and spread more quickly. Breast cancer is given a grade of 1 to 3, with 1 the least serious and 3 the most serious.

cancer stage: how much cancer is present in the body and whether it has spread. Doctors use a system of letters and numbers to describe how much cancer has spread.

cell: the basic unit of which all living things are made.

chemotherapy *(KEY-mo-THAIR-uh-pee)***:** treatment with drugs that kill cancer cells.

diagnosis *(die-ug-NO-sis)***:** identifying a disease by its signs and symptoms, and by using imaging tests, laboratory tests, or biopsy. For most types of cancer, a biopsy is needed to be sure of the diagnosis.

external beam radiation therapy: radiation that is focused from a source outside the body on the area affected by the cancer. It is much like getting an x-ray, but at a higher dose. Radiation to the breast can be delivered from outside the body in different ways.

fatigue *(fuh-TEEG)***:** bone-weary tiredness that often doesn't get better with rest. It is different from being tired because of not having enough sleep. It is feeling as if your brain, body, and emotions are all tired. Fatigue is one of the most common side effects of cancer treatment.

flap procedure: breast reconstruction in which a doctor uses tissue from somewhere else in your body to make what looks like a breast. The tissue can come from your abdomen, back, or buttocks.

gene: a segment of DNA inside a cell that has the information to make a specific protein. Genes are responsible for traits passed on in families, like hair color, eye color, and height, as well as susceptibility to certain diseases.

genetic counseling: the process of counseling people who might have a gene that makes them more susceptible to cancer. The purpose of the counseling is to help them understand what genetic test results might mean, help people decide whether they wish to be tested, to explore what the test results might mean, and to support them before and after the tests.

genetic testing: tests performed to determine whether a person has certain gene changes known to raise cancer risk. Such testing is not recommended for everyone, but for people with specific types of family history. Genetic counseling should be part of the process.

hormones: chemical substances released into the body by the endocrine glands like the thyroid, adrenals, or ovaries. Hormones travel in the blood and set in motion certain body functions. Testosterone and estrogen are examples of male and female hormones. Some kinds of breast cancer need hormones so they can grow.

hormone replacement therapy (HRT): taking hormones after you have gone through menopause, when your body stops making hormones. Also known as postmenopausal hormone therapy (PHT).

hormone therapy: cancer treatment that interferes with hormone production or action. This is not the same as hormone replacement therapy (HRT) that may be used after menopause. Hormone therapy also may involve surgery to take out hormone-producing glands. Hormone therapy may kill cancer cells or slow their growth.

insurance benefit: the medical care, drugs, and supplies covered by health insurance.

intraoperative radiation therapy (IORT): a type of external beam radiation in which one large dose of radiation is given in the operating room after the tumor is removed but before the wound is closed.

lumpectomy *(lump-ECK-tuh-me)*: taking out a cancerous lump and some of the breast tissue around it, but not the full breast. Also called *breast-conserving surgery*.

lymph nodes *(limf nodes)*: small, bean-shaped collections of immune system tissue like lymphocytes, found along lymph vessels. Lymph nodes help fight infections and also have a role in fighting cancer, although cancers sometimes spread through lymph nodes. Doctors may remove some lymph nodes to find out whether there is cancer in them.

lymphedema *(LIM-fuh-DEE-muh)*: a complication in which lymph fluid collects in the arms, legs, or other part of the body. This can happen after the lymph nodes and vessels are removed by surgery, injured by radiation, or blocked by a tumor that slows normal fluid drainage. Lymphedema can happen even years after treatment and can become a life-long problem.

malignant *(muh-LIG-nunt)*: cancerous; dangerous or likely to cause death if untreated. Compare with *benign*.

mammogram *(MAM-uh-GRAM)*: an x-ray picture of the inside of your breast. Mammograms are done with a special type of x-ray machine used only for this purpose. *Screening mammograms* are used to help find breast cancer early in women who don't have any symptoms. *Diagnostic mammograms* help the doctor learn more about breast lumps or other breast changes.

mastectomy *(mas-TEK-tuh-me)*: surgery to remove all of the breast (or both breasts) and sometimes other nearby tissue.

menopause *(MEN-uh-paws)*: when a woman's menstrual cycles stop. During this time, hormone levels typically fluctuate before they stabilize at much lower levels. Menopause usually takes place in a woman's late 40s or early 50s, but it can also be brought on suddenly by surgical removal of both ovaries (oophorectomy), or by some types of chemotherapy that destroy ovarian function.

metastasis *(meh-TAS-tuh-sis)*: when cancer cells break away and spread to other, distant parts of the body, often by way of the lymph system or bloodstream.

monoclonal *(MA-nuh-KLO-nuhl)* **antibodies:** special immune proteins made in a lab and put into the body. Monoclonal antibodies can be used to treat cancer. Some can attach to parts of cancer cells to either affect the cells directly or mark the cells so they can be found and attacked by the immune system. Other monoclonal antibodies are attached to chemotherapy drugs and deliver these treatments directly to the cancer cells, killing them with little risk of harming healthy tissue.

nausea: an uncomfortable, queasy feeling of the stomach that may make you feel like vomiting.

nipple reconstruction: a type of breast reconstruction where tissue for the nipple and areola is taken from a patient's body, usually from the newly created breast or, less often, from another part of your body. Tattooing may be used to match the nipple of the other breast and create the areola.

oncologist *(on-KAHL-uh-jist)*: a doctor with special training in the diagnosis and treatment of cancer.

palliative *(PAL-ee-uh-tiv)* **treatment:** treatment that relieves symptoms, like pain, but is not expected to cure the disease. Its main purpose is to improve the patient's quality of life. Sometimes, chemotherapy and radiation therapy are used as palliative treatments.

pathology *(path-AHL-uh-jee)* **report:** a report that explains the type of breast cancer you have, how big the tumor is, and its grade. Doctors write the report based on what they see when looking at the tissue under the microscope. They use the report as a guide to help plan how to treat your cancer.

patient assistance programs: programs that offer free or lower-cost medicines to people whose prescription drugs aren't paid for by insurance.

prognosis *(prog-NO-sis):* a prediction of the course of your disease and an estimated outlook for survival.

prosthesis *(pros-THEE-sis):* also called a breast form. It is padding shaped like a breast or part of a breast that can be worn in your bra to fill it out after breast surgery.

protein: a large molecule made up of a chain of smaller units called amino acids. Proteins made by your body help it grow, fix itself when it's hurt, stay healthy, and do other important things.

radiation therapy: treatment with high-energy rays (like x-rays) or particles (like protons) to kill or shrink cancer cells. A special machine is used to point x-rays at the cancer to kill or hurt cancer cells (external beam radiation); sometimes radiation is given by putting radioactive material into the body where the cancer was located (brachytherapy or internal radiation). See also *brachytherapy, external beam radiation therapy, intraoperative radiation therapy, palliative treatment.*

recurrence: to happen or occur again, like cancer that comes back after treatment.

remission: when tests don't show any cancer after treatment. Cancer appears to be gone.

risk factor: anything that is related to a person's chance of getting a disease such as cancer.

sentinel lymph node biopsy *(SEN-tin-uhl limf node BY-op-see)*: a procedure involving the removal of the first lymph node (or nodes) to which cancer cells are likely to spread from the primary tumor. In some cases, there can be more than one sentinel lymph node. For this procedure, a radioactive substance and/or dye is injected into the tumor, near the tumor, or in the area around the nipple. The substances or dye will collect in one or more lymph nodes, which are then removed at surgery and examined for the presence of cancer cells. See also *lymph node.*

side effects: unwanted effects of treatment, like losing hair because of chemotherapy or feeling tired from radiation therapy.

supplement: a vitamin or mineral that doesn't come from foods but comes in pills, for example.

targeted therapy: treatment that attacks a part of cancer cells that is different from normal cells, as opposed to the treatment that harms all cells. Targeted therapy sometimes works when standard chemotherapy drugs do not, and these therapies tend to have fewer side effects than chemotherapy.

tissue *(TISH-oo)*: cells that work together to perform a particular function.

tumor *(TOO-mer or TYOO-mer)*: an abnormal lump or mass of tissue. Tumors are sometimes cancer (malignant) and sometimes not (benign).

x-rays: low levels of radiation that make a picture of the inside of the body, as in mammograms. High levels of x-rays can be used in radiation therapy to kill cancer cells.

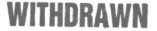

WITHDRAWN

31901059912032